The care and management of mentally disordered offenders poses a major challenge to criminal justice agencies and psychiatric services. These patients, 'the people nobody owns', are particularly vulnerable to political and professional change, and, as psychiatric services become increasingly community based, the task of meeting the needs of the offender, as well as expectations of public protection, becomes a more difficult prospect.

This book brings together the papers and a summary of the discussion presented at a Cropwood Round Table conference organized by the Institute of Criminology and the Department of Psychiatry of the University of Cambridge. Seeking to define future needs and directions in legal and service provisions, it includes perspectives from the fields of criminology, sociology and social psychiatry, as well as contributions from practitioners and administrators.

Remarkable for the tenacity and depth with which the expert contributors address the problems, this volume will be essential reading for all professionals working in the psychiatric and criminal justice systems with this frequently marginalized client group. Through a searching examination of the situation within one jurisdiction, it points the way to service developments, improved care management and new research opportunities that have universal applications.

T0275667

THE MENTALLY DISORDERED OFFENDER IN AN ERA OF COMMUNITY CARE: NEW DIRECTIONS IN PROVISION

THE MENTALLY DISORDERED OFFENDER IN AN ERA OF COMMUNITY CARE: NEW DIRECTIONS IN PROVISION

Proceedings of the 20th Cropwood Conference,
10–12 January 1990

Edited by
WILLIAM WATSON and ADRIAN GROUNDS

Institute of Criminology and Department of Psychiatry, University of Cambridge

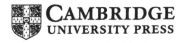

CAMBRIDGE
UNIVERSITY PRESS

CAMBRIDGE UNIVERSITY PRESS
Cambridge, New York, Melbourne, Madrid, Cape Town, Singapore, São Paulo

Cambridge University Press
The Edinburgh Building, Cambridge CB2 2RU, UK

Published in the United States of America by Cambridge University Press, New York

www.cambridge.org
Information on this title: www.cambridge.org/9780521403429

First published 1993
This digitally printed first paperback version 2006

A catalogue record for this publication is available from the British Library

Library of Congress Cataloguing in Publication data
Cropwood Round-Table Conference (20th:1990:University of Cambridge)
The mentally disordered offender in an era of community care: new directions in
provision: proceedings of the 20th Cropwood Conference, 10–12 January 1990, Institute
of Criminology and Department of Psychiatry, University of Cambridge / edited by
William Watson and Adrian Grounds.
    p. cm.
ISBN 0-521-40342-1 (hc)
1. Criminals – Mental health services – Great Britain – Planning – Congresses.
2. Prisoners – Mental health services – Great Britain – Planning – Congresses.
I. Watson, William, 1953– . II. Grounds, Adrian. III. University of Cambridge.
Institute of Criminology. IV. University of Cambridge. Dept. of Psychiatry. V. Title.
[DNLM: 1. Community Mental Health Services – congresses. 2. Forensic Psychiatry –
congresses. 3. Mental Disorders – congresses. 4. Prisoners – psychology –
congresses. HV 8841 C948m]
RC451.4.P68C76
365′.66 – dc20 92-48693 CIP

ISBN-13 978-0-521-40342-9 hardback
ISBN-10 0-521-40342-1 hardback

ISBN-13 978-0-521-03339-8 paperback
ISBN-10 0-521-03339-X paperback

Contents

Conference participants

Dr D. Bennett
Emeritus Physician, Bethlem Royal and Maudsley Hospitals, London, UK.

Mr R. Baxter
Assistant Secretary, C3 Division (Mental Health), Home Office, London, UK.

Mr W. Bingley
Legal Director, National Association for Mental Health (MIND), London, UK.

Mr L. Blom-Cooper
Chairman, Mental Health Act Commission, London, UK.

Prof A. Bottoms
Director, Institute of Criminology, University of Cambridge, UK.

Dr P. Bowden
Consultant Forensic Psychiatrist, Bethlem Royal and Maudsley Hospitals, London, UK.

Mr D. Brown
National Association for the Care and Resettlement of Offenders (NACRO), London, UK.

Mr M. Carroll
St Mungo's Housing, London, UK.

Dr D. Chiswick
Consultant Forensic Psychiatrist, Royal Edinburgh Hospital, Scotland, UK.

Dr T. Craig
Director, National Unit for Psychiatric Research and Development (NUPRD), London, UK.

Mr I. Crowe
Lecturer in Criminology, University of Sheffield, UK.

Mrs S. Dell
Research Associate, Institute of Criminology, University of Cambridge, UK.

Mr N. Dholakia
Commission for Racial Equality, London, UK.

Ms H. Edwards
Assistant Director, National Association for the Care and Resettlement of Offenders (NACRO), London, UK.

Dr A. Fowles
Lecturer in Social Policy, University of York, UK.

Mr E. Francis
Director, Afro-Caribbean Mental Health Association, London, UK.

Dr A. Grounds
Institute of Criminology, University of Cambridge, UK.

Prof J. Gunn
Professor of Forensic Psychiatry, Institute of Psychiatry, London, UK.

Miss M. Hancock
Social Services Inspectorate, Department of Health, London, UK.

Dr C. Hedderman
Home Office Research and Planning Unit, London, UK.

Dr K. Herbst
Policy Development Officer, Mental Health Foundation, London, UK.

Dr A. Holland
Consultant Psychiatrist, Bethlem Royal and Maudsley Hospitals, London, UK.

Dr P. Joseph
Senior Research Fellow, Institute of Psychiatry, London, UK.

Mr C. Kaye
Chief Executive, Special Hospitals Service Authority, London, UK.

Mr M. Lee-Evans
Consultant Clinical Psychologist, AMI Kneesworth House Hospital, Royston, Hertfordshire, UK.

Mr B. McGinnis
Policy Director, Royal Society for Mentally Handicapped Children and Adults (Mencap), London, UK.

Mr E. Packer
Honorary Secretary, Outer London Justices' Clerks' Society, London, UK.

Mrs E. Parker
Secretary, Mental Health Act Commission, London, UK.

Prof E. Paykel
Professor of Psychiatry, University of Cambridge, UK.

Dr J. Peay
Lecturer in Law, Brunel University, Uxbridge, Middlesex, UK.

Mr F. Powell
Head of Nursing Services, Special Hospitals Service Authority, London, UK.

Mr H. Prins
Lately Director, School of Social Work, University of Leicester, Leicester-shire, UK (Conference Chairman).

Dr J. Reed
Senior Principal Medical Officer, Department of Health, London, UK.

Mr V. Rees
Principal, Priority Care Division, Department of Health, London, UK.

Ms J. Renshaw
Director, Good Practices in Mental Health, London, UK.

Dr G. Robertson
Lecturer in Forensic Psychiatry, Institute of Psychiatry, London, UK.

Mr J. Shaw
Branch Crown Prosecutor, Crown Prosecution Service, West Mercia, UK.

Dr G. Shepherd
Top Grade Clinical Psychologist, Fulbourn Hospital, Cambridgeshire, UK.

Ms L. Sinclair
Legal Director, Royal Society for Mentally Handicapped Children and Adults (Mencap), London, UK.

Mr G. Smith
Chief Probation Officer, Inner London Probation Service, London, UK.

Mr J. Stanford
Director, Legal Studies, Board of Extra-Mural Studies, University of Cambridge, UK.

Mrs W. Start
Magistrate and Mental Health Review Tribunal Member, Nottingham, UK.

Dr P. Taylor
Director of Medical Services, Special Hospitals Service Authority, London, UK.

Mr J. Walker
Chief Inspector, Leicestershire Constabulary, UK.

Prof N. Walker
Institute of Criminology, University of Cambridge, UK.

Mr W. Watson
Graduate student, Faculty of Social and Political Sciences, University of Cambridge, UK (Rapporteur).

Prof D. West
Institute of Criminology, University of Cambridge, UK.

Mr J. Westall
Policy Officer, National Schizophrenia Fellowship, Surbiton, Surrey, UK.

Judge D. West-Russell
Chairman, Home Secretary's Advisory Board on Restricted Patients, London, UK.

Prof J. Wing
Director, Research Unit, Royal College of Psychiatrists, London, UK.

Prof Sir John Wood
Professor of Law, University of Sheffield, UK.

Dr R. Wool
Director, Prison Medical Service, Home Office, London, UK.

List of tables and figures

Figures

Preface

The care and management of mentally disordered offenders poses a major challenge to criminal justice agencies and psychiatric services. As psychiatric services become increasingly community based rather than hospital based, the task of meeting the needs of the offender, as well as expectations of public protection, becomes a more difficult prospect. Public disquiet about the care of the chronically mentally ill in the community and about the protection afforded by mental health legislation has been voiced. Difficulties are experienced by the police and courts in securing psychiatric care for mentally disordered offenders, and the severely mentally ill are over represented in the remand prison population. Inadequacies in current provision for mentally disordered offenders in Britain are a matter of current concern in both the Home Office and the Department of Health, who have recently carried out a wide ranging review of services for such individuals (Department of Health/Home Office, 1991).

This book brings together the papers and a summary of the discussion presented at a Cropwood Round Table Conference, organized by the Institute of Criminology and the Department of Psychiatry, University of Cambridge, in January 1990. The purpose of the conference was to consider future needs and directions in legal and service provision for mentally disordered people in the criminal justice system. A distinguished group of participants representing a wide range of interests attended the conference, and the papers included perspectives from the fields of criminology, sociology and social psychiatry, as well as contributions from administrators and practitioners.

The significance of the conference was threefold. First, contemporary research and service developments in social and community psychiatry were brought to bear on the field of forensic psychiatry. To date, the framework of forensic psychiatry services and mental health legislation has been primarily hospital based. New thinking is required to move beyond this, as the major gap in provision for mentally disordered offenders is now in the community. It is therefore important to take account of the lessons and insights that have emerged from recent work in social psychiatry, and we were fortunate that several of the major figures in the development of social psychiatry and new services for the long-term mentally ill in Britain contributed to the proceedings. Secondly, the conference was held against the immediate background of the publication, shortly beforehand, of two White Papers outlining Government policy for a fundamental restructuring of hospital and community services, namely the White Papers on the reform of the National Health Service, which is now being implemented, and on Community Care (Department of Health, 1989a; 1989b). Thirdly, the range of statutory agencies, non-statutory agencies, and academic disciplines represented at the conference was unusually wide. The constituency of people with a concern about mentally disordered offenders extends far beyond the confines of the small professional field of forensic psychiatry. Mentally disordered offenders are a marginalized group whose members move in and out of numerous spheres of influence, including the courts, the police, prisons, probation and social services, NHS hospitals and services, and charitable organizations. This theme is encapsulated in the title of the opening paper 'Offender-patients: the people nobody owns' by Herschel Prins who chaired the conference proceedings throughout.

The remaining chapters are divided into three groups. The first group of papers by Dr Douglas Bennett, Professor Sir John Wood and Dr Jill Peay, provides a critical appraisal and overview of possible future directions for general psychiatric services and for mental health law. Dr Bennett emphasizes the irreversible move towards community psychiatry, and characterizes the groups for whom more sophisticated, specialized services need to be developed. Professor Sir John Wood discusses the impact of legal reform, particularly as enshrined in the Mental Health Act 1983, on psychiatric practice. He argues that legal powers cannot in themselves ensure that resources and professional attitudes facilitate the flexible movement of individuals between various levels and types of care. Dr Jill Peay then examines, from a criminological perspective, the framework of legal provision for mentally disordered people in the criminal justice system, and she challenges the validity and justice of having two rigidly separate systems for mentally disordered and non-disordered offenders.

The second group of chapters comprises a series of perspectives on service needs. Dr Tony Fowles and Dr Paul Bowden both critically examine the alleged relationship between rising prison populations and declining patient populations in psychiatric hospitals. Dr Fowles' examination of available statistics casts doubt on the theory that there is a major transcarceration of population from mental hospitals to prisons, and Dr Bowden argues that those chronic psychotic people who do end up in prison could not be engaged in treatment elsewhere without a wholesale return to large scale detention in closed hospitals. A change in policy is therefore required in order to improve conditions and facilitate the provision of treatment for the mentally ill in prison.

Professor John Wing's chapter on defining need and evaluating services succinctly outlines the principles of investigation which might be applied in research on specific services for mentally disordered offenders. Recent, exploratory studies of the experience of black people in magistrates' courts and forensic psychiatry services are described in the chapter by Mr Deryck Browne, Mr Errol Francis and Dr Iain Crowe. They raise important wider questions about issues of race, and emphasize the need for ethnic monitoring and further research in this field.

The next three chapters examine the needs of mentally disordered offenders from the viewpoints of the probation service, the prison medical service and the courts. Mr Graham Smith specifies ways in which the probation service can contribute in the management of such offenders, and reveals the considerable scope that exists for closer and more effective liaison between criminal justice agencies and psychiatric services. Dr Rosemary Wool discusses the problems of achieving diversion of mentally disordered prisoners to hospital, and outlines the Prison Department's policy for providing for those mentally disturbed prisoners who remain in the prison system, a policy that includes a role for specialized prison establishments. The degree to which inappropriate remands in prison custody can be prevented by diversion at an earlier stage is considered in Dr Philip Joseph's chapter, in which he describes his innovative psychiatric assessment service located in two magistrates' courts in London. The scheme facilitates hospital admission, results in discontinuance of criminal proceedings in over one-third of cases, and his findings suggest that this way of deploying psychiatric resources in court could have a substantial impact in reducing the numbers of mentally disordered defendants remanded in custody. This pioneering project is now being emulated more widely in the United Kingdom.

The last set of chapters focuses on the planning and implementation of new styles of service. Mr Mike Lee-Evans gives an illuminating account of the recent growth and future prospects of private sector hospitals, whose rapid development has been a consequence of the shortfall in provision for patients perceived as 'difficult to manage' in local NHS facilities. The emphasis in Dr Geoff Shepherd's chapter returns to the community, and he provides a rigorous, critical review of the concept and practice of case management, a model which is prominently proclaimed, but with insufficient definition and analysis, in the Government White Paper on Community Care (Department of Health, 1989*b*). The final chapter in this section, by Dr John Reed, provides an account of the development of policy in the Department of Health towards provision for mentally disordered offenders. The paper anticipates the themes that have since emerged in the Department of Health/Home Office Review which emphasizes the need for flexible, responsive services and transfers between facilities according to clinical need (Department of Health/ Home Office, 1991). A final concluding review by William Watson highlights some theoretical and research implications raised by the conference proceedings.

The main chapters are followed by short summaries of the themes that emerged in discussion. We have generally avoided verbatim transcripts of individual comments for two reasons: first, the discussion sessions in the conference extended over nine hours, and the amount of text had to be kept within reasonable bounds; and secondly, we wanted to ensure that the conference participants could engage in debate, unconstrained by concern about attributed statements appearing in print. Instead, we have sought to select and highlight what we perceived to be the main ideas and links between the papers that emerged in the discussions.

Finally we would like to express our gratitude to Maureen Fry, Caroline Gaskin, Helen Platt and Helen Ruddy for all their secretarial help in preparing the manuscript; and to the Barrow and Geraldine S. Cadbury Trust, the University Department of Psychiatry and the Nuffield Foundation for their generous financial support for the conference. Our particular thanks to Herschel Prins and Wendy Start whose interest and support helped sustain the project from its outset to its completion.

William Watson   Adrian Grounds
Toronto   Cambridge

Part I
Introduction

1

Offender-patients: the people nobody owns

H. PRINS

Introduction

When my fellow conference organizers prevailed upon me, not only to act as chairman for this discussion of future provision for mentally disordered offenders but, in addition, to make some introductory observations and to sum up our deliberations, I can only assume they did so in the knowledge that I am something of a 'meddler' – a bit of a 'Jack of all trades and master of none'. I suppose this role has some merit since it enables me to survey some aspects of the scene with a degree of detachment. It certainly enables me to make some brief comments on the legal, psychiatric and administrative aspects of the problem, to ask some questions, but not necessarily provide any answers. If I do no more than raise our consciousness of some of the issues, hopefully this will provide a background for some answers that may emerge as a result of the contributions from the distinguished speakers who are to follow me in the next two and a half days. Maybe my role can best be likened to that of 'chorus' or 'prologue' used to such good effect by writers such as Shakespeare. Unfortunately I cannot aspire to the heights of imaginative puissance of the 'brightest heaven of invention' deployed by chorus in *Henry V*. Such talents as I have may be likened more to those of the plodding, ancient Gower in Pericles, who sings 'a song that old was sung' (Act I). I hope, I shall, at least, be unlike the worthy Gower and cause 'no din but snores the house about' (Act III). Nor, hopefully, shall I be like Dryden's Midwife, who 'laid her hand on his Thick Skull, with his Prophetick blessing – Be Thou Dull.' *Absalom and Achitophel* (Pt.2 476).

Offenders, deviants or patients?

When I made my first substantial foray into the social aspects of forensic psychiatry I called my book Offenders, *Deviants or Patients?* (Prins,

1980). I did this because I felt that not only was there ambivalence, uncertainty and ambiguity about the people who constituted my title, but that the title also reflected a constantly shifting mad, bad and sad group, whose madness, badness and sadness were also present in ever-changing degrees within perhaps the same individual. These were the people who nobody really wanted to know; they were, as my late friend and colleague Dr Peter Scott used to say, the 'not nice' patients. I have come to describe them to my audiences as the 'unloved, the unlovely and the unlovable'. Of course, some of these offender-patients do stimulate our interest because of the nature of their crimes (some of them quite horrific). We must therefore be very careful not to obtain vicarious satisfaction from their misdeeds for I would venture to suggest that the boundaries between their behaviour and our own are not perhaps so great as we sometimes like to imagine (Prins, 1988, 1990). And, of course, some of them also present a challenge because we are in the business of trying to prevent the repetition of further mayhem (Prins, 1988). Those mentally disordered offenders who tend to present as 'social nuisances' rather than as 'social menaces', are, in fact, as Hajioff (1989) has recently pointed out, probably the least attractive to most psychiatric and allied professionals. Often dull, unresponsive, lacking in personal graces of any kind, they do not present as very endearing clients or patients. I hope that I have said enough already to indicate that, although we shall be looking at a number of the psychiatric, legal and administrative barriers that may stand in the way of an effective and co-ordinated service for mentally disordered offenders, there is a very real need to examine our own attitudes and not hide defensively behind them by projecting them on to others.

A brief glimpse at the international scene

There is always a tendency to think that the 'grass is greener on the other side of the tracks' and that other countries have found the solution to providing resources for, and managing, this difficult and demanding group of patients. A recent special issue of the *International Journal of Law and Psychiatry* on *Forensic Administration* (Vol. 11 (4), 1988) carried a series of articles describing the situation in Canada, USA, Holland and Scandinavia. In all these countries there are reported difficulties. There are accounts of problems caused by over- and under-centralization, by unilateral policy decisions that seem to take no account of the population being served (sounds familiar!) and of funding problems.

The most helpful pattern appeared to exist in Scandinavia, because, as I understand their particular provisions, every citizen seems to have a basic right to all kinds of health services irrespective of status, penal or otherwise. Maybe this is a phenomenon we should examine more carefully to see what lessons could be learned.

Some comments and questions

I now wish to make some comments and raise one or two questions that hopefully will help to facilitate our receptiveness to the expert contributions that are to follow. I have divided them, quite arbitrarily, into two headings: *Legal* and *Psychiatric and Administrative*; of course they both overlap. My observations are to be viewed as preliminary sketches for a canvas to be painted upon in much more detail by others.

Legal

Do the provisions of the existing law serve to help or hinder provision? A few somewhat random illustrations must suffice (as they are the subject of detailed comment shortly). We know that whether an offender receives psychiatric or a penal disposal often seems somewhat arbitrary. From the defendant's point of view it often appears to depend upon who your judge was, the constitution of the jury (if a jury trial of say diminished responsibility was involved), the quality of your counsel and the credibility of your psychiatrist. Certainly the current arrangements for dealing with pleas of diminished responsibility seem to result in unedifying contests between the legal and psychiatric professions. It is sad that what appeared to me to be sound proposals to amend the law relating to murder, have, if you will forgive the phrase 'died the death'. At an entirely different level of operations, the 1983 *Mental Health Act* was hailed (as was its predecessor) as a landmark in the care and protection of the mentally disordered. (For accounts of its genesis see Bluglass, 1985; Roth, 1985.) Founded on civil libertarian views, but tempered to some extent by psychiatric reality, the Act has in my view proved to have certain inherent weaknesses. (It has certainly given the lawyers a 'field-day', or a number of 'field-days'; there have been more judicial reviews in five years than in the entire existence of the 1959 Act.)

Rightly or wrongly, it now appears to be more difficult to detain some people compulsorily for treatment – particularly the mentally impaired. I can foresee a time (perhaps too gloomily some might say) when we may witness a reversion to the days before the passing of the 1913 *Mental Deficiency Act*, when you will recall the defectives (as they were then called) were to be found in large numbers in our prisons. It is certainly my impression, having talked to probation officers and local authority social workers countrywide, that there are very real worries that this group of highly vulnerable people are landing up in the penal system and look like continuing to do so, though as we shall see tomorrow, there is a need to examine the figures with care. (For a recent account of some of the difficulties in implementing community care and the steps taken in one city – see Bean & Mounser, 1989.) Relationships with central government, especially the Home Office, do not seem to have been made any easier under the new legislation. For example, the mental health review tribunals now have no power to make formal recommendations for a transfer in restricted cases (see also Wood, 1985). The increase in legal representation in all categories of cases (surely a good thing in itself) has led, for a variety of reasons, to some serious delays in tribunal hearings and lack of movement through the system. Now that tribunals have been given power to discharge restricted patients, one may also ask about their relationship with the Home Secretary's Advisory Board on Restricted Patients. It is therefore particularly helpful that Judge West-Russell, Chairman of that Board, is with us, as well as departmental officials. It is also pertinent to observe that he is also here as a senior representative of the judiciary.

Psychiatric and administrative

There seems little doubt that there appears to have been an increasing reluctance on the part of psychiatric professionals to work with offender-patients in recent years. Scannell (1989) has summarized many of the reasons for this, and these are too familiar to this audience to bear repetition. However, one reason that may be important, and that seems to have received rather less attention, is that psychiatric professionals find it harder to work together than is often recognized publicly. Because of this there are undoubtedly 'demarcation' disputes. In this context it is worth remembering that lawyers, doctors, nurses, psychologists, and social workers are all trained in different ways and acquire different role models and perceptions. It is therefore hardly surprising that offender-patients may often end up as 'pigs in the middle' and as readily available vehicles for the projections of the professionals involved in the management of their cases. Coupled with this, is the continuing climate of nihilism in the treatment of offenders and offender-patients. Psychiatrists and others seem to be reflecting this attitude in the view held by some of them that, for example, psychopaths should no longer be managed in the hospital system. (See Grounds, 1987; Dell & Robertson, 1988.) At an administrative level, the provision of resources, if they can be said to exist at all, has been piecemeal. Since the abolition of the Board of Control by the 1959 Act, provision for the mentally disordered in general seems to have received all too little central focus and direction. By this I mean that it is all too easy for a small and highly vulnerable group to become submerged in the totality of health care provision. The setting up of the Mental Health Act Commission has done something to help to redress the balance. The Griffiths Report (1988) and the recent White Paper *Caring for People* (DHSS, 1989a) certainly provide opportunities for us to think in new ways about resources. However, funding is still likely to be a key problem unless we are able to break out of existing modes and models of thought and attempt to look at the problem anew. How might this be achieved? In the next two and a half days we all have an unusual opportunity to try to think afresh. Perhaps we need to look at new (and perhaps controversial) ways of funding and entitlements to it. For example, should funds 'travel' with the offender-patient? Would this help to obviate the demarcation disputes that so frequently frustrate us and block progess? Perhaps this is also the time to break down boundaries. It may be that for far too long we have allowed the very complexity of the problem to obscure our vision. Because many offender-patients, as I have already suggested, are unlikeable and unresponsive, they are for this very reason especially vulnerable to political and professional 'climatic' changes. Thus, they can easily disappear from professional view. All this is particularly important at a time when our society has become increasingly ethnically diverse and when we are happily becoming rather more sensitive to the needs of other particularly vulnerable groups such as female offenders. I hope that we shall also pay especial attention to the needs of the mentally handicapped during our discussions. All of us at this conference, whether as formal speakers or as participants, have an obligation to widen our horizons, and, as I have said, to embrace new ways of thinking. Only in this way, as it says in the Book of Isaiah 'shall the eyes of the blind be opened and the ears of the deaf be unstopped' (xxxv, 5–6). If we do not try to think afresh, we are merely continuing to heap disadvantage upon an already disadvantaged group. I began these brief remarks by describing myself as 'chorus' or 'prologue'. The remainder of my duties are hopefully a mixture of kindly 'minder' and perhaps accoucheur to the effects of your combined creativity.

Part II

Future directions for psychiatric services and mental health law

2

Future pattern of psychiatric services

D. BENNETT

Yesterday

Having been told to speculate on the future of psychiatric services, I remembered that there was a time when psychiatrists were presumed to have a crystal ball in the cupboard, as well as a trick cycle in the back yard. Those happy days were before society saw psychiatrists as the psychiatric fuzz or more recently as unnecessary jacks of all trades. Never effective with my crystal ball I decided to follow the advice of Aneurin Bevan who said 'why study the crystal ball when you can read the book?'. With this advice it is my intention to scan the book of the past as a possible guide to the future. Certain themes persist and since change is slow, it seems possible that one can predict what may be happening at the beginning of the 21st century.

Let me begin at the end of the First World War when there was public unease about the ways in which the mentally ill were detained: a general fear that the whole system of lunacy administration was wrong and that widespread cruelty existed in public mental hospitals. A Royal Commission on Lunacy and Mental Disorder was appointed and reported in 1926 when it spelled out ideas which have guided change in public mental hospital psychiatry since that time (Home Office, 1926). The Commission's report stressed the close relationship of psychiatry to general medicine, the need to reduce legal intervention in the detention of the mentally ill and the need to secure care for the discharged patient. It recommended that local authorities could spend more to establish out-patient services and that the connection between psychiatry and the Poor Law should end. This seemed to mark the beginning of the end of the isolation of psychiatry from medicine and of the mental hospital from the wider community. Psychiatry could develop as a medical 'scientific' subject and play a part in medical education.

Psychiatrists at that time hoped that early treatment both inside and outside the mental hospitals would diminish patient chronicity. *The Mental Treatment Act* 1930 followed the Commission's report and made voluntary treatment available for many patients. But the Poor Law was not finally abolished until 1948.

At the end of the Second World War the National Health Service came into being. It was important for psychiatry that the same salaries were paid to psychiatrists as to physicians and consultants in other specialities. It also brought all hospitals, the general or mental, whether formerly managed by local authorities or voluntary bodies, under the same regional and national direction. In theory at least 'mental hospitals had equality of status before the law with other hospitals and an equal share of the financial cake' (Hill, 1969). So psychiatric patients for the first time in history were to be treated like all other patients. Other aspects of the Welfare State were also important, in particular those elements of the insurance system which gave the sick person monetary benefits making it easier for such people to support themselves, and for their families to care for them outside hospital, without the financial disadvantages which had existed under the Poor Law.

Later, further changes detailed in the *Mental Health Act* 1959 made it easier for patients to enter or discharge themselves from hospital without legal intervention. There was a recognition of the trend towards community care, and from this time, the long-stay population in mental hospitals began to decline; there were more admissions but patients stayed a shorter time. Neuroleptic medication was introduced in about 1955. Combined with the other social changes that were taking place, it helped to reduce psychotic behaviour and to restore control of perceptual disorders in some patients.

The chronic long-staying population of mental hospitals has continued to decline in numbers. The individual hospitals showed surprisingly similar rates of decline and this reduction has, according to Leff (1986), shown no sign of levelling off. Much of the uniformity is due to mortality. Between 1976 and 1986 about 18 000 patients who had stayed more than five years were taken off the rolls of mental hospitals; 6000 were discharged but 12 000 died. This long stay population is no longer being replaced in such numbers. There have been many other changes, but the most significant seems to have been the White Paper on Hospital Services which confirmed the integration of psychiatry in medicine when it indicated that improvements in treatment and care made it possible for all psychotic patients to be treated in district general hospitals (DHSS, 1971*a*).

Today

So if we look at the position today we see that we are at the end, or almost at the end, of a psychiatry isolated in mental hospitals many of which are in the process of being closed. Psychiatry is increasingly integrated into medicine; the mentally ill individual is no longer treated as a pauper lunatic but is admitted to a general hospital psychiatric unit or treated in his own home as a mentally ill patient.

Clinically there have been significant changes in treatment, and advances with new medications, psychotherapy, family therapy, day services, rehabilitation and employment services have played their part. Local district services are slowly replacing admission to asylums, while new hospital developments, for those still requiring 24-hour supervised hospital care, have been developed (Wykes, 1982).

This has had beneficial effects; institutionalism is avoided, patients have a better quality of life, while being treated more considerately and preserving their dignity. There are however, disadvantages for those patients who are unable to care for themselves adequately, have no family, or who show seriously deviant behaviour. The current *laissez-faire* outlook of some professionals and some members of the public means that such patients may not be admitted to a psychiatric unit or, because of their unco-operative behaviour, may be deemed unsuitable patients and not detained.

There has been growth in specialized psychiatric care with increasing knowledge and expertise. We now have services for people with phobias; with anorexia nervosa; for adolescents and students in distress; for marital problems and sexual disorders. There are psychiatrists interested in post-traumatic stress reactions after disasters or the victims of torture. There are services for those who have broken the law, who are dependent on alcohol or habit forming drugs, are elderly, or immigrants and those with epilepsy and brain diseases.

Social services seem to be retiring from the psychiatric scene. Social workers were potent interdisciplinary workers until 1970 when they took over the management of their own departments and soon after were swamped by the outcomes of the Maria Caldwell affair. Since then they have become ever more absorbed with the problems of child abuse which dominate their work.

Psychiatrists are not too interested in the unromantic and undramatic area of chronic illness. The late Henry Miller felt that the need to concentrate resources on the care of the aged and handicapped would demand the ruthless sacrifice of those frills which interest the best doctors. These challenges had no appeal for him, nor do many young psychiatrists espouse rehabilitation.

The increasing number of psychologists only make a relatively small contribution to the work of rehabilitating chronic patients, although there are important exceptions. In spite of more realistic appraisals of the limitations of behaviour therapy, they are more interested in modifying anxiety while only a few attempt to assess patients' disabilities or to shape the environment to help adaptation.

As these and other professions eagerly assume new responsibilities, interprofessional rivalries will influence the necessary co-operation between disciplines and what effect this will have within or without the health service is difficult to foresee.

At present we are in an awkward period of change. Although mental hospitals have been running down for 30 years or more, we have never fully faced the implications of their closure. Now the House of Commons Social Services Committee (1985), the Audit Commission (1986) and the Griffiths Report (1988) have all made suggestions for rationalizing the methods of allocating and paying for 'packages of care'. Community care for the elderly and disabled has been equated with community psychiatry for the mentally ill in spite of their differences, although some objections to this seem to have been recognized. The care of patients is being forced into the market place where it must be cost effective and managers seem to be working with these aims in view regardless of the needs of patients. One cannot visualize units competing to treat the most disabled. A Cinderella service, always deprived and still deprived, needs generous treatment more than managerial 'efficiency'.

Tomorrow

Without fear of contradiction I can say that the fundamental disabilities of people with schizophrenia or manic-depressive psychosis have not improved over the years. How we care for these sufferers has improved their secondary disabilities significantly: we have stopped making them worse. But I suspect that we shall have the same severe problems to cope with in the next decades. We cannot hope for the possibility of simple chemical or psychological cures. Although biological psychiatry is trying to stage a renaissance, one must doubt the possibility of its successful parturition. Improvements in social psychiatry are possible, but since these require the interaction of social events and clinical events and the social events are caused by other people, this is not easy.

Greater emphasis will be placed on the individual in his family and in his social context, although it is difficult or impossible to prevent the occurrence of life events. But support from people in the community, as well as from professionals and other patients is helpful and will receive greater attention. We know that discharged long-stay patients do not want to return to hospital and that a very large majority of their relatives share that opinion (Johnstone *et al.*, 1984). Psychiatrists in this country are free to work outside hospital and, if they can work in a multidisciplinary team, they will be in a good position to form a therapeutic alliance with relatives or other carers; this will in some cases prove an alternative to hospital admission or in other cases will use hospital admission as part of a more constructive plan.

It may seem that the Poor Law is dead, but is it? A half a mile or so from the Maudsley Hospital there was an institution where 'under one roof were being performed the functions of an old people's home, a lodging house for the itinerant labourer, alcohol rehabilitation centre, half-way house for the discharged prisoner and perhaps a dozen other functions besides' (Edwards *et al.*, 1986). Griffith Edwards was speaking of the Gordon Road Reception Centre (now closed) but he might have been speaking of many mental hospitals which look like the work houses or the prisons that they were. They are disappearing and their old patrons are leaving. Their service will be sought by fewer and fewer patients, but I am less certain that we have severed our link with the Poor Law in human terms. Those inadequate and rootless wanderers that form a 'stage army' marching from doss house to prison and on to mental hospital and back again are not as some would have us believe, the result of psychiatry's or the mental hospital's abrogation of their responsibility. The House of Commons Social Services Select Committee (1985) said of them that 'they long ante-date community care policies'.

In the years ahead there will be less discussion of the burning contemporary issue of community versus hospital care. We shall instead begin to develop a community psychiatry which we still lack and which is frequently being discredited before it has arrived. Instead, the argument will be about the nature of the community care and particularly the division between those conditions which are seen and treated by the primary carers and those which are the responsibility of the specialist caring services. More attention will be given to the needs of the majority in primary care who respond to treatment, but the expansion of that service will depend very much on the national financial situation. More attention will also have to be given to the inadequate and rootless wanderers. They can probably be divided into three groups who require services which do not yet exist on an adequate scale.

First there are patients with 'challenging behaviour' who are likely to be a danger to themselves of others, who have had a history of violence, who have been compulsorily detained or have been in a secure unit in the past two years. Of the 246 very old, very long-stay patients in Cane Hill Hospital on the 31 March 1988, 16 showed this challenging behaviour, but the rehabilitation and resettlement teams for those three London health areas served by the hospital do not believe that a regional solution is needed nor do they accept the idea of 'haven' care. They are planning to place them with other persons who have not been long-term hospital patients, but who have similar needs in specially built units within the hospital grounds or in the 24 hour highly supported homes outside the hospital (NUPRD, 1989). Such people are frequently rejected by today's hospitals, sometimes justifiably because they cannot be detained under current mental health legislation; sometimes for more cynical reasons.

We shall continue to have a big job to do for a second group of individuals who 'cope inadequately' because they do not have the skills to care adequately for themselves, or the motivation to do so, or relatives or people to help them. For these patients both immediate care and continuing care will be needed. Anxieties are expressed by the public about the conditions of single men who live alone in hostels and community homes. The public raise questions about adequate care when they see stained shirts, cigarette stubs on the floor and a lack of sheets and blankets on the bed. The disabled people themselves are sure of one thing: they do not want to return to hospital where they cannot do what they want to, when they want to do it. If there are relatives, what they want is more help from the extramural services and not more mental hospital care (Creer & Wing, 1974). Even if these disabled patients are well adjusted or adapted to life in the community it is always possible that they will break down, and if we are to avoid the ensuing difficulties they need emergency services on 24 hour call every day of the year. These services must be able to respond rapidly, within a half hour, to calls from their relatives or other people who are having acute psychiatric problems and who need help from the services. We also need continuing care teams which stay in continuing contact with a group of well-recognized chronic patients who have persistent difficulties with behaviour, lack of skill or lack of motivation. They will have to be based on a key worker or a case management system and they will have to adopt an assertive approach, not waiting to be asked or to be called, but, on their own initiative, see that patients are washing themselves and eating, as well as receiving their medication. Such care can be undertaken without staff being intrusive (Hoult, 1986). It is as effective as what might be achieved by more coercive mental health legislation although some slight revision of the law might be anticipated. We also need other facets of an integrated, flexible support system such as day centres, work and, for those with no families or families who will not or cannot help, we need various kinds of accommodation.

Finally there are those people who are called by Oxford's Elmore Community Support Team the 'difficult to place'. In other words, agencies of various kinds find these people difficult because they do not fall within the responsibilities of one single agency. Usually they show a combination of bizarre or disruptive behaviour, homelessness, problems of general health, alcohol or drug abuse, offending and mental disorder. Three-quarters of them have criminal records. In Oxford there are at any one time about 150 such people who are not expected to improve. Two-thirds of them are mobile transients, but a third of them have their roots in Oxford. Between the units in any large network of services, such as exists in that area, there will be gaps and it is in those gaps that the Elmore project operates. The team is made up of three support workers; a community psychiatric nurse, a social worker, and a co-ordinator. The support workers do not stress their training, and the organization avoids being regarded as a resource. They feel it must remain flexible and able to negotiate with other agencies. Thus, the staff are in a position to share out tasks or different parts of the service which an individual needs and which is offered by the whole network. They can relieve any one service of having to provide residential services or day care, financial resources and so on and neither the police, nor probation, nor landlords, nor social service departments have total responsibility for that individual. They are supporting the service almost as much as they are supporting the individual (Vagg, 1987).

The care of patients with dementia will almost certainly move out of the psychiatric hospital and be more closely linked with the care of the more physically handicapped geriatric patient. It seems that in the care of the elderly mentally infirm, as in the care of the mentally abnormal offender, the alcoholic and other groups, we shall see a tendency on the part of psychiatric services to limit 'direct service' to the patient or client and to expand 'indirect service' through collaboration and consultation with other caretakers and care givers. This trend will in part be determined by the limitations of psychiatric manpower. While there has been an explosive increase in the numbers of psychiatric staff – not just psychiatrists – in recent years, there are still not enough people to meet the growing burden which others are eager to thrust on to the psychiatric professions. For this reason I believe that day treatment in one form or another will continue to expand.

Finally, the position of the mentally disordered individual will continue to change. In the past 50 years such people have secured the right to be treated as patients, rather than as persons of unsound mind and have been freed to a certain extent from legal constraints and from the stigma of institutional confinement and pauperism. More recently there has been concentration on their civil rights, which are no longer compared with those of the physically ill, but with the rights of the average citizen. This is all to the good if such rights can be obtained without a danger of neglecting the seriously deviant client: it is a difficult balance.

Psychiatry has ceased to be a purely professional concern; it has 'gone public' and a considerable body of laymen consider psychiatry to be not only a matter of professional but of public interest. There are more television and radio programmes, more Parliamentary interest and a significant heightening of the salience of mental illness in terms both of overt political activity and broader social awareness. This will continue and develop and in the future I think users of the services will be increasingly active.

Discussion

The recognition that 'community care has lost its innocence' (Turner, 1988) pervaded the debate arising from Dr Bennett's paper. Three main themes were prominent. First, it is necessary to unpack the meaning of the concept of community care; secondly, it is time to move away from regarding hospital and community as polarized alternatives; and thirdly, there are unresolved questions about the extent to which the functions of the traditional hospital can be replaced in community settings, particularly for patients whose behaviour is chronically disturbed or provokes public alarm. In addition, the situation of the mentally handicapped was discussed.

The concept of community care

In a number of important respects community care is undoubtedly desirable. Providing care for mentally disorderd people outside the mental hospital allows them freedom to make their own decisions; and the aim of restraining people's lives no more than is necessary in order to deliver the treatment process is clearly right. As Dr Bennett remarked, one can properly talk only about quality of care in mental hospitals, not quality of life. To have quality of life people must be able to make their own decisions.

However, in the community the distinction between treatment and setting must be understood. In many cases, patients are offered a planned treatment experience but an unplanned placement experience. They may be placed in situations in which professional agencies are not competent to deliver what the clients need in order to sustain their quality of life. This is well recognized by those who argue for the retention of hospital-based asylum care, and who claim that patients may be discharged from an environment where at least they have a roof over their heads and friends and some sort of support, to another environment in which they have none of those things; where they are homeless, financially destitute, have no support, and may be vulnerable to exploitation and victimization.

The antithesis between hospital and community

Productive discussion might be facilitated by avoiding the antithesis between hospital on the one hand and community on the other. Instead, a positive agenda of clinical objectives should be specified itemizing what is wanted. Then questions about settings can be considered, for example whether particular neighbourhoods have the capability of providing care or whether this has to be delivered. We probably require both hospital and community care, but the kinds of hospital may be very different from those we have known in the past.

Questions were raised about the extent to which attitudes, working practices and contractual arrangements inhibit health service staff from implementing properly based community care. The bulk of staff are still staying in the hospitals, and the traditional provision of out-patient clinic appointments may be less useful than the capacity to provide rapid psychiatric assessment and treatment at the patient's location. The roles of clinicians and the nature of treatment differ when delivered outside hospital: they have to change in order to suit the routine of the patient's life.

Agencies outside the statutory psychiatric and social services may doubt whether this is being achieved. From their perspective, the integration of psychiatry with other hospital-based medical services can appear as an off-loading of responsibility for the long-term mentally ill to other non-specialized agencies, and the range of non-medical functions that were provided by traditional mental hospitals may not be replaced in a specific and organized way by these other agencies. Psychiatric services have retained a core of more treatable and acceptable patients, and some of the more chronically disabled are left to others outside the NHS. Occasionally, such agencies may develop, on their own initiative, innovative and successful projects for the mentally disordered. For example, St Mungo's Housing in London, a charitable organization for the homeless, has developed residential projects for psychiatric patients, using untrained staff. Such developments may, however, be unconnected with wider frameworks of planning and liaison.

It was argued that, in the case of secure provision, perimeter security was needed to protect society against the dangerous mentally disordered offender, but that conditions within the perimeter tended to be over-secure. Staff want to feel psychologically safe and to have the authority of the key in the pocket. But this may be incompatible with maximizing choices for the patient within the institution.

Community care for the severely disturbed

Questions have yet to be resolved about the extent to which community based psychiatric services can meet the needs of more severely disturbed patients. There are two alternative models for dealing with people with severe behavioural problems. One approach is to place them, together with others who have 'special needs', in a specific unit; and the second model is a 'rescue service' whereby a team travels to the patient's location in order to intervene, and then goes away. The idea of delivering treatment to people where they are without inflicting unnecessary changes to their life experience is attractive, but will it work for those whose behaviour is persistently disturbed? Public attitudes also have to be taken into account. The visible presence of homeless people who are obviously mentally ill, for example may exacerbate public fear of crime in that neighbourhood.

The relation between the needs of the criminal justice system and provision of community care has to be considered. At present, by default, some 'community care' is provided by the penal system. Those working in the criminal justice system would not regard prison as part of community care, although some working in the health service may regard it in this way. Some remand prison settings function in effect as acute psychiatric wards. Seriously mentally ill people who ought to be in hospital go to prison. The catchment area hospital knows that they should be in hospital, but lacks the facilities to take them. From the perspective of agencies in the criminal justice system, hospitals do seem necessary as the starting point for meeting the needs of mentally disordered offenders. Community care may be the ultimate objective but is unlikely to be where treatment will start.

However, the scenario outlined by Dr Bennett does not include services which explicitly provide some kind of containing and controlling function for the mentally disordered whose behaviour is unacceptable in the community, even though there is a public expectation that psychiatric services will provide such a function. The degree to which this can be successfully done in community-based services needs to be established. It may be the case that people now working in psychiatric services are unwilling to resume the controlling and containing function. There has been a major change during the last generation in the way nurses see their roles, and outside specialist secure provision there is less willingness to regard the containment of behaviour as a primary part of the nursing role. In the future, clinical staff will need to overcome their reluctance to accept that in some cases containment is necessary, and it need not be seen as symbolic of failure. Only when this attitudinal barrier is passed is it possible then to consider the development of constructive therapeutic programmes for those small groups of mentally disordered people who do need a degree of containment.

The needs of the mentally handicapped

The above issues need to be considered in specific relation to mental handicap. Usually the needs of the mentally ill 'lead' thinking about service development. The relevance of new proposals to mental handicap can not be simply assumed, but requires separate examination. Are the principles governing provision the same or different? There is a tendency to find excuses for not dealing with chronic patients, and mental handicap might be regarded as the most chronic of conditions. Mr Brian McGinnis,

Policy Director of the Royal Society for Mentally Handicapped Children and Adults (Mencap), succinctly summarized the approach which, in his view, should prevail.

'... people with mental handicap need to be treated as individuals and helped to grow and develop and choose in a setting and among a range of opportunities which are no more abnormal than their individual support needs from time to time require. Support and independence need to be held in balance: the first without the second lacks point; the second without the first lacks substance. Because we believe in a needs-led rather than a theory-led service, we are more concerned with the quality of people's lives in those settings where they are at present than with relocation as an end in itself. One of the most disturbing features of the present developments in services is that we may be busy designing structures and systems none of which fits the requirements of people who have *inter alia* or on its own, something we can legitimately call a mental handicap. If prisons are geared to a rehabilitation or punishment process, hospitals and NHS units to a treatment process, and community care facilities to a social development process, designed in each case by people who know little or nothing about mental handicap for people who don't have a mental handicap, the allocation process is doomed to failure, however good it is.'

3

Future directions for mental health law

J. WOOD

Introduction

Before attempting to assess the shape and effectiveness of the current law relating to mental health, attention has to be given to the purpose and impact of regulation by law. In modern society, with increasing concern for individual 'rights', it is inevitable that the treatment of the mentally ill should be more closely regulated by law. It is nowadays unfashionable to believe that good sense and benevolence are alone satisfactory safeguards where society attempts to aid disadvantaged sectors of the community. Many feel that 'caring' has dangers that arise from inbuilt conservatism and smugness. With hindsight it has become clear that each generation has either unquestioningly embraced some terrible procedures or has espoused reforms in the name of treatment or social policy that have later been seen to be serious mistakes (see Scull, 1989). The inadequacies of the professions and their frequent inability to react quickly to criticism and to review with open minds their own practices are equally clear. One of the current solutions to these failures is the belief, now prevalent, that much of the former bad practice can be eliminated and future mistakes avoided by 'the law'. Reliance is placed upon legal rules such as the Mental Health Act 1983 and formal avenues of challenge such as the mental health review tribunals. These provide a now well understood system but one that is not without some lack of clarity.[1]

It must be said at once that it is very naive indeed to believe that 'the law', despite its majesty, does not inevitably have its own weaknesses and creates, in turn, its own problems. Its role is in need of similar, if not greater, scrutiny to ensure that its own methods of providing safeguards do not suffer from the same atrophy or lack of self awareness and thus fail to be sensible and effective. Above all, legal regulation must not be mistaken for the system itself, when it is merely the safeguard. 'Regulation by law' is both a concrete description of a body of rules enshrined in statute and case law and an indication that a particular area of activity is governed and regulated in a special way. Such regulation has an important and distinct character from which many consequences flow, of which some – such as the establishment of a relatively reasonable and clear set of rules of conduct, or the provision of an easily accessible forum to challenge what is being proposed or done – are undoubtedly beneficial; whereas others – such as the central role given to the thinking and habits of lawyers or the diversion of attention and resources to the secondary business of considering challenges – are usually found to be a mixed blessing. This is clear from the almost inevitable tensions that arise between many of the professionals working in the area regulated by law and the lawyers themselves.

Two aspects of legal regulation fall to be examined; the legal framework itself,[2] after several years, merits critical appraisal, as does the way in which the rules operate in practice, especially those aspects which call for the intervention of lawyers by way of forensic challenge. But first some critical attention has to be given to the impact of greater emphasis on the law as regulator of the care and control of the mentally ill.

The impact of legalization

In many subtle ways the nature of the practices that have become subject to legal regulation will of necessity change, solely to meet the new demands of the legal approach. The law brings into play attitudes developed over the ages by the legal system, attitudes often developed in many disparate fields of legal activity such as criminal trial, civil disputes and property transactions, which impose a special approach and logic. A great deal that arises from this is advantageous, indeed essential – the lawyer's insistence on clarity, on rules properly made and consistently adhered to, for example – but there is much else which sets up tensions and distortions – the concentration upon 'words' rather than the underlying reality is the most pervasive example and the tendency to model everything upon the adversarial approach the most destructive. There is a tendency on the part of lawyers to see every problem as having 'two sides'.[3] This is not only a staggeringly ignorant simplification, especially where sensitive social relationships are concerned, it also tends to hinder the settlement of problems, for the adoption of an adversarial approach encourages each 'side' to put its 'best' case forward and then concentrates attention upon the differences, thus tempting 'the parties' to unwise exaggeration and even, in some cases, destructive stubbornness.

To be fair, regulation by law is most successful where the matters with which it is concerned are clear, concrete and generally accepted. Unfortunately there is much in the sphere of mental health which is not merely less than clear, it is the subject of fierce controversy within the professions concerned, or between those professions. To look to the law to clear up these difficulties is either to seek to impose one's own view of matters by way of legal regulation, or to ask the law to arbitrate in disputes of a specialized and highly technical nature, a task for which it has few, if any, qualifications.

Finally, attention has to be drawn to the limitations within which the law works. It will tend to be formulated having regard to the resources which are available and its application will certainly be limited if appropriate resources are absent. This is a considerable limitation upon effectiveness. It is not merely a question of the overall size of those resources; it involves the much more difficult question as to their type. The Victorian and Edwardian period left a massive infrastructure of hospitals and beds, which for very many reasons are no longer regarded as a major resource and are being gradually phased out, to be replaced by more modern methods of containment and control for mental patients thought to need them. The legal structure has to adapt, as far as it can, to such major changes in the attitude to acceptable methods of nursing and supervision.

Legal framework

The general principles of the present framework were put in place in 1959 and amended in 1983 and there seems to be general satisfaction with the current legal framework amongst practitioners, if not amongst theorists. There appears to be little pressure for root and branch reform but there are undoubted practical problems which merit attention and improvements that can be suggested.

Some trends, however, are in need of careful assessment. First, and probably most important, is the impact which legal control of professional workers may have on their work and attitudes. The imposition of a legal system has two generally damaging effects. It creates tension if professionals feel constrained to an extent which seriously inhibits their professional judgment. It may also lead to a bureaucratic approach which stifles the best, who wish to carry out their work with speed, energy

and efficiency. It must not be forgotten that the work of the Mental
Health Act Commission is a major 'control' over those caring for the
mentally ill, less obviously adversarial than the mental health tribunals
but nonetheless likely to heighten these effects.[4]

What follows is a selection of some points where there appears to be
need for fresh thinking and perhaps reforms. It is by no means exhaustive.

Definition of mental disorder[5]

Although it has been the subject of considerable disagreement in the past,
the classification of the categories of patient to fall within the Mental
Health Act seems to be now fairly stable and generally accepted. What is
obvious and wrong, however, is the haphazard way in which both the
psychopath and the mentally ill are identified and brought within the
hospital system.

Admission

It is a matter of serious concern that it is by no means certain that a
psychopath will be detained by a court in a mental hospital, rather than in
prison. It is even more obvious, from the streets, that seriously mentally
ill persons are not necessarily cared for in a hospital or home. The
destination of a mentally disturbed offender seems to be very much a
lottery, depending upon many factors such as the individual's willingness
to raise the issue of his mental state in court and the assessment of the
appropriate order made by the judge. There are two philosophies on the
appropriateness of compulsory detention in hospital, but this cannot
justify lack of consistency.

Additionally, although there are many types of detention involving
psychiatric supervision such as a prison with a hospital wing, a special
psychiatric prison such as Grendon Underwood, the special hospitals, the
regional secure units and a hospital with some secure accommodation or
indeed without, movement between them is not a common feature of the
present system, and is not incorporated in the legal powers of tribunals. It
is unlikely that a sentencing judge will be able to choose with certainty the
best environment to contain the prisoner he is dealing with for the future
and it is clear that the system does not efficiently ensure that the
individual finds the correct 'level'.

The matter is utterly confused by the attitude of the psychiatric profession to the concept of psychopathy and the criminal justice system's need to deal with the 'dangerous' individual thought likely to re-offend and so in need of detention longer than the normal 'tariff'. Its own partial solutions – preventive detention and extended sentences – obviously failed and the willingness of the psychiatrists to undertake long-term 'treatment' as a medical problem, offered an apparently neat solution that the sentencing practice could not effectively cope with. No wonder it was eagerly welcomed. After considerable criticism, the view is increasing that psychopathy is both hard to identify and not anyway a problem with medical content (Clare, 1980). The potential withdrawal of psychiatrists as a profession and the likely disappearance of more and more prisoners with damaged personalities, who are potential recidivists, into prisons will serve to hide one of the key problems faced under the Mental Health Act, and if it is not accompanied by special provisions in the prison service, which seems very unlikely, the underlying problem of 'abnormal' re-offenders will remain without answer.

Discharge

The lottery of uncertain diagnosis and lack of clarity about appropriate places of detention leads to many clear examples of injustice. An individual chosen for detention in mental hospital is denied a set date of discharge, which may indeed be brought forward for good conduct, in return for the onerous task of convincing others that there is a favourable prognosis and it is safe for him to enjoy more freedom. It is an exceptionally difficult task, for opinions as to future conduct are inevitably highly subjective.

Perhaps the most serious obstacle to fair discharge is the impact of public opinion. The person who leaves prison and re-offends may attract public criticism but this will be directed to the law, whereas a released patient who re-offends brings criticism, often most vociferous in character, on the mental health review tribunal system with the possibility of affecting future cases adversely.

Transfer

The powers of a mental health review tribunal are limited to discharge and do not extend to transfer. This limitation appears to arise from the proposition that no consultant should be obliged to admit a patient to his care. The logic, based on the great importance of the doctor—patient relationship, is clear and the rule rarely attracts discussion yet it exerts a very powerful influence on the management of patients. Viewed objectively this is undoubtedly a very serious weakness in the structure of the system, especially where the patient is in the hospital of greatest security. The length of the wait for transfer has been little short of scandalous in many cases – periods of five years and over not being unusual.[6] It is surely a principle at the heart of the legal rules on mental illness that the patient should be constrained only as long or as much as is essential for his health and for the well-being of the community. This would seem to require, as an essential, transfer from one level to the next, in either direction and 'on trial' or more permanently.[7]

There are basically three layers of provision – secure hospital, open hospital and community care, but each has many variants and so there is considerable possibility of uncertainty. For example, the regional secure units have neither a clear place in the heirarchy nor a character that is easily described, since they vary considerably in their admission policies and treatment regimes. Their creation appeared to add a much-needed step between special hospital and ordinary hospital but many who have done well at the special hospital have their progress hampered because there is an additional step which prudence, rather than judgment, dictates should be taken before fuller freedom. The varying nature of these units, which should have added to the hospital services available, becomes a disadvantage if geographic considerations are the chief determinants of placement.

Hospital and community care have been greatly changed over recent years, a process that will continue. Again the theoretical gain to patients of flexible choice is being diluted by lack of resources and of clarity about what is precisely available. For example, many modern psychiatric units in general hospitals are plainly designed for relatively short stay patients. The transfer problem for those who need longer term care has been a growing weakness very obvious to tribunals denied the right to order transfer.

There is too an underlying lack of clarity in the law, as a recent case shows.[8] A restricted patient, found not to be suffering from one of the qualifying states of mind, was held to have properly been discharged but also made subject to recall. Once the basic qualifications for the imposition of an order are no longer present then it should, logically, be discharged and further problems, if they arise, dealt with afresh. The decision is paternalistic, and though in some ways none the worse for that, runs counter to the civil liberties view of the statute.

Management

It was inevitable that the legal mind would want to test the medical assumption that containment in, say, a special hospital without any 'medical treatment' was permissible.[9] This point had, however, been anticipated in the legislation which defined medical treatment to include nursing, care, habilitation and rehabilitation.[10] It has to be acknowledged, despite this, that such a wide definition blurs the essential distinction between treatment and containment and adds to unease that the system is built on unclear distinctions or that apparent safeguards for the patient or public are discretely concealed.

There has been a tendency of the tribunals to attempt to 'manage' the patient through the use of adjournments to await the result of treatment or to see if a suitable transfer could be arranged. This has been challenged by the Home Office who see the tribunal's job to adjudicate, not to exercise some form of continuing control.[11] The courts have taken this view too. Adjournments, it has been made clear, are permissible to await a report of, for example, a recent course of treatment but not to allow a reconvening after a period to see how things have gone. The dispute is not quite so important as it seems since with the possibility of annual appeals a patient is usually able to ensure a following tribunal in a matter of months.

It should not be overlooked that legal representatives of certain patients do lend their weight to such pressures, often seeking adjournments, unwarranted though this may be. This management by the patient's solicitor denies the patient his right to appear before a tribunal which may have advantages even where there is no discharge.

Some specific issues

The various powers of the tribunals give rise to a number of difficulties which are now well known enough to enable a brief indication to suffice.

Section 2, Mental Health Act 1983

The introduction of the right to challenge detention immediately after compulsory admission was a notable advance – from the tribunal viewpoint, the most important change of the 1983 Act. It has led to a considerable work load. The time scale for hearing the appeal was inevitably tight – the detention runs for only 28 days and for a tribunal to have an impact it should be operative in the tenth to twentieth day. This is in fact what has happened and it is to the credit of the tribunal administrators, the hospital staff concerned and the lawyers who represent the patient and have to take sketchy instructions. The question has to be asked – how effective are such tribunals?

The statistics show that they have some point. The periodic statistics issued by the regional offices show a variation in discharge rates of between one in 4–5 and one in 10. Bearing in mind the very short period covered by the discharge – at most 15–20 days – the cost effectiveness is questionable. That is not to say some check is not appropriate, merely that the full tribunal, which can hardly operate with its usual approach since the evidence is sketchy and partial, might be replaced by a simpler procedure.

It is necessary for there to be a very detailed study to see precisely whether the system could be streamlined in some way. This point is made because there seems to be very little evidence of patients being detained under these rules without any justification whatever or in error. The safeguards that surround detention appear to be very effective. There is a very apparent keenness on the part of the social workers concerned to ensure that the patients' interests, in terms of civil liberties, are fully taken into account. That means that the tribunal is most often called to make a difficult decision in those cases where the patient has, as a result of medical treatment and a few days of hospital care, made a quick improvement. Should there be a discharge of the order or would a further period be legally justified? is the key question. There is not a lot of indication that patients are deliberately detained for the whole period without good reason. The value and cost effectiveness of s.2 tribunals will no doubt one day be examined and perhaps less formal checks instituted in their place if the facts so warrant.

Indeed, the only obvious point of misuse is that in several cases it appears that a patient, with a history of admissions, often under order, is first detained again under s.2 where a s.3 order appears to be more logical.

Section 3, Mental Health Act 1983

There is a very important problem for the patient who has been detained under s.3. In many cases the well-being of the patient in the community depends upon the continued acceptance of medication. One of the actions taken by consultants has been to retain the order whilst letting the patient live at home. A recall to hospital to renew the order might be all that is required of the patient who is complying with the consultant's wish that treatment be accepted from the nurse at home. The most obvious advantage of this procedure is that where a patient shows signs of a relapse, or starts to ignore his treatment, then a recall can be quick and easy whereas the rules governing re-admission, in the attempt to protect, require a marked breakdown before a new order can be made. The consultant, who has knowledge of the patient, would prefer to take up more intensive treatment earlier than is likely from such re-admission procedure.

Despite this undoubted benefit a lawyer is bound to challenge the paternalism of such action. Neither is it surprising that the courts have taken the view that the 'long leash' is not permissible under the current legislation.[12]

The result is that a debate has arisen about whether a community treatment order should be introduced into the legal code of control of patients. There are, it will be appreciated from what has already been said, good arguments in its favour, since it would offer another level of control of a patient, less onerous than the others.

There are worries that will undoubtedly be put in opposition. Paternalistic supervision tends to assume that what the professionals are insisting upon is good for the patient, whose views cannot be effective in opposition. In some instances it may be that the patient should be allowed some choice, accepting a lesser quality of life rather than treatment. It is equally possible that a patient may feel that the consultant's care has turned to conservative inertia or to a level of drugs that is excessive and destructive of the quality of life. Over-protection of the patient is to many as much a breach of civil liberties as detention in hospital. It is a matter which should be extensively debated.

The role of the tribunal in determining challenges against such community treatment orders would have considerable difficulties. If a recall of a patient, made subject to a community treatment order, were to be allowed perhaps before or perhaps immediately after recall, then the tribunal will find itself playing a significant role in the admission of the patient – a new departure that needs careful consideration. So far, the mental health review tribunals have played no part in admission, and they should only be given this role reluctantly. It is also doubtful whether the reason for recall is truly justifiable since the reason for non-compliance with treatment will be clear and what remains in issue is the necessity for recall which is likely to turn largely upon previous patterns of behaviour in some cases or likely deterioration if medication is stopped for a lengthy period in most of them. Tribunals, as a body, may be reluctant to undertake a task where the issue is so difficult to resolve, it being substantially one of attitude to the extent to which paternalism is justified. Perhaps a less stringent criterion for re-admission would be preferable.

General matters

There is no pressing need for a major reform of the law and no strong pressure either, except perhaps for a number of relatively minor matters.[13] This is perhaps right, since the greatest improvements will undoubtedly be achieved by greater administrative efficiency, that seems almost as difficult to secure. Some of the needs can be briefly set out as examples.

(*a*) As more types of care become available, in both the hospital and the social services, it is important that the individual patient can move as easily as possible from one level to another. Facilities have to be available at each level to meet the needs of patients and to give those charged with caring for patients ready access to other levels of care for the patient. Those charged with legally checking that civil liberties are not infringed must also be given greater opportunity to discharge their obligations sensibly and to the benefit of the patient. Where the choice is a stark one of maintaining or discharging the order, the work can only partially be done.

(*b*) There needs to be attention given to the number of controls imposed upon doctors and hospitals, and some check on their frequency of use. The patient's position may be reviewed by the Mental Health Act Commission, the hospital managers and the mental health review tribunals. Although the tasks of the Commission and the tribunals to some extent overlap, there is a fairly clear distinction between control of the medical aspects of detention and the civil liberties aspects. There is little co-ordination, however, and the effect may be disturbing or disruptive to patient care. The role of the managers is much more obscure, and apparently fitfully used.

Neither body seems aware of the other and the patient is likely to be confused by two appeals, of rather different character, following each other within a short time and apparently with no co-ordination.

(c) It is perhaps time to reconsider the exact purpose of tribunal review. In theory it is to decide the narrow question, is the detention justified by reference to the legal criteria? In practice where discharge is very unlikely indeed there is an inevitable tendency to disrupt the detention itself. Should the right to appeal be controlled, especially in the early years of the psychopathic offender?

The frequency of tribunals is an important aspect of this problem, especially in respect of restricted patients. The restricted patient is in some sense serving a sentence – although many would deny this. Nevertheless, in a large number of cases, especially where the diagnosis is psychopathy rather than mental illness, time served plays an important part in the decision to recommend transfer or to release. If this point is valid two consequences have to be faced.

First, the patient who has committed a serious crime will have little chance of an early release. What effect should this have on tribunal hearings in the early years? The reasonable answer 'none' raises the spectre of hearings at which the possibility of a favourable outcome is remote so the proceedings must have an unreality about them. When release was the prerogative solely of the Home Secretary, at least everyone knew that the tribunal had a major function to perform, that of adding to the Home Secretary's store of information and opinion upon which the decision to move the patient on would eventually be made. Although in theory the tribunals still perform this function, it is barely openly recognized, and would be better expressly laid on the tribunal.

It can also be argued that once the notional tariff for the offence that has led to hospital detention has been passed the patient is entitled to expect a very rigorous consideration of his plea for release. In many ways, the longer a patient remains in a secure hospital the more difficult it is for him to convince others that he is a safe risk. Particularly with sex offenders, the result is, perhaps rightly, extreme caution and often very lengthy detention. The caution, however, may be said to be oppressive if no limited trials, with greater freedom are readily available. In general terms they are not. This failure to provide a well-organized system of trials, with return to hospital automatic if things do not go well, is one of the abiding weaknesses of the system, even though some improvement may be detected, at least by the optimists.

Conclusions

The debate as to the quality of our present legislation on mental health and the detention of patients is, at its roots, a philosophical debate on which there is a considerable amount of literature. In extreme positions are those who would leave most of the power to the professional judgment of psychiatrists with limited rights of appeal to obviate serious misjudgment and those who favour giving the most limited role to compulsion and seeking stringent rules to justify detention only where the patient or the community are at serious risk. As always with 'political' matters, the practical solution must lie in a compromise and compromises are difficult to achieve, hard to maintain and police, and above all vulnerable to swings in general attitudes to the underlying principles of the permitted limits of restraint on freedom.

It is important, especially at a time when a system has developed a rhythm and momentum of its own, to identify the areas where greater clarity, or new thinking is required.

The basic medical concepts

Underlying the whole system is the opinion and esteem in which psychiatry itself is held. It is a sad fact that some of the psychiatry concerned is uncertain at best and at worst strongly contentious. Mention has already been made of changing attitudes to psychopathy, the category of mental abnormality which has been the basis of diverting offenders from the criminal justice to the hospital system and has provided a significant number of long stay detainees who have absorbed a great deal of medical and legal attention. Doubts about the underlying concept inevitably destabilize practice and encourage strong legal challenge to detention, which, in turn, fosters the adversarial approach.

Similar clarification is required as to the problem of mental impairment. It is inevitable that the mentally impaired will raise dilemmas of a different nature to those of mental illness or psychopathy. The border-lines between some types of impairment and mental illness are not clear. It is important to offer clear forms of care that vary to match different needs.

Resources and administration

The legal system is only as good as the resources available to it and the ability to use those resources effectively. It is the part of the system which is hardest to change or use effectively. At the present time, there is a great deal of flux and it is here that the greatest difficulties arise. The great mental hospitals are closing; community care of a wide range of diversity is being created – a very welcome but extremely slow process; regional secure units have been created, though more are needed, whilst the imaginative Eastdale Unit attached to Rampton Hospital has been unaccountably closed; the psychiatric units in general hospitals offer a much improved service but appear to adapt badly to the medium stay patient. Such comments can be extended but the underlying point is clear. There needs to be a clearer range of treatment available. Above all, and this point should perhaps be written in capitals, movement between the various levels and types of care should be easy. It is here that all the worst aspects of professional and administrative thinking seem to militate against the hapless patient.

It is difficult to recommend legal reform to break some of these well-known bottle-necks since powers of transfer do not guarantee that resources will be available for their effective use and the patient may find such an imposed transfer raises resentment.

Admission

The current legislation seeks to provide sound safeguards against un-necessary or thoughtless compulsory detention. Although there is con-siderable unease about its effectiveness the detailed research fails to convince and tends to lead to proposals that would, in seeking to protect some against detention, leave many who need care to remain without the help that is available.

Many of the suggestions for reform – to abolish the role of the nearest relative for example – are difficult to support. The danger is that such reforms tend to arise not wholly from concern for the patient. They also involve the role of the professional. For example, the approved social worker often adopts a quasi-judicial function but it would be wrong to institutionalize this as no professional, whose expertise is part of the decision, can properly be called on in this way.

Crime and detention

Much of this paper has been concerned with patients coming from the courts. The problems here are many – the concept of psychopathy, the frequency and effectiveness of tribunals and above all the lack of clarity between the civil route to detention and the criminal.

Particular issues

There are numerous issues, many of which are much debated, that require resolution. Most pressing is the community care order because the sufferer from schizophrenia who can exist in the community for long periods but is subject to periodic breakdown is a common problem. It is important to devise a sensible and relatively fair procedure to help ensure continued medical care in the community yet allow re-hospitalization at an early stage to avoid a damaging breakdown.

Another topic of frequent discussion is the greater use of guardianship. It has been so well rehearsed that there is really no excuse for inaction. As usual, the real obstacle is that there is no certainty that effective guardians are available and thought needs to be given to that aspect of the problem.

It is impossible to cover comprehensively the whole range of improvements and reforms of the system that have been raised in the literature. As the wind swings between paternalistic care on the one hand and civil liberties and due process on the other fine tuning becomes necessary. It is also necessary to meet changes in medical theory and practice and, more regrettably to match realistically the legal and medical actions to the resources available so as not to raise unfulfilled expectations. The general verdict must surely be that the system initiated by the Mental Health Act 1959 has proved to be fundamentally sound. The time is close for reconsideration and review to secure improvement. There is, however, a fundamental danger that too great a concern with the system at work may divert attention from the central issue – that the aim is effective and humane treatment and care of those with mental disability.

Discussion

The discussion of Professor Wood's paper focused on pressing practical and ethical issues confronting the relationship between the law and psychiatry. These concerned three specific and related areas: Professor Wood's concern that psychiatry had become marked by self-doubt and clinical timidity; the possibility of clashes between professional groups, and especially between medical and legal forms of practice, not viewed here as an intrusion of medical concepts into the legal system, but as an intrusion of legal notions of responsibility and redress into established patterns of therapeutic practice; and a set of more detailed practical issues facing the mental health review tribunal system.

The problem of clinical timidity

Professor Wood outlined his view that the psychiatric profession is in a phase of major self-doubt and timidity. This has caused a problem for the criminal justice system, which had been relieved to have some recidivists labelled as psychopaths and placed in the special hospitals, thus dealing with the problem of determining the tariff for frequent offenders. With psychiatrists increasingly uncertain about the existence and treatablity of psychopathy, and of their capacity to cater for these individuals, enormous problems have been created for the system, and for the tribunals in particular. Equally, psychiatrists, who primarily see their work as involving care, have become uncertain about facilitating the long-term control of individuals. Professor Wood also drew attention to the way in which this clinical uncertainty may have led to unfortunate variations and inconsistencies in the national pattern of provision. The regional secure units may be taking patients from the special hospitals that the tribunals would have previously discharged into the community, creating difficulties for the tribunals in interpreting their duties. It was his opinion that some ex-special hospital patients may find intensive group therapy situations within the RSUs very difficult to cope with.

It was argued that psychiatry was uncertain because society was uncertain about psychiatry; society had spent a long time telling psychiatrists that they ran 'cuckoos' nests', and that they should eschew control. It was also pointed out that psychiatrists should not be given the task of dealing with recidivists for the benefit of the legal system, and that if indeterminate sentences within the criminal justice provisions were required, these should be introduced by the Government. Professor Wood accepted that society has asked for the locks to be removed from open hospitals, and that these hospitals therefore no longer have the facilities to deal with difficult incidents. He also accepted that the certainty with the psychopathic diagnosis applied by psychiatrists had been enthusiastically accepted by others primarily because it seemed like the solution to the insoluble problem of intractable recidivism.

Multi-disciplinary provision

Several contributors commented on the problems experienced when a number of professions combine to deliver a system of provision. It was pointed out that some of the problems experienced in placing mentally disordered offenders in suitable settings arose through the reluctance to accept them expressed by nurses rather than doctors. It was suggested that nurses may feel they lack the resources and possibly the skills to deal with difficult patients. Nurses needed to take a more professional approach to these issues, it was suggested. It was recalled that at one time, and before the development of modern forms of medication, nurses working in wards catering for difficult individuals had a high level of morale and commitment, even if their work was little valued by outsiders. This attitude needed to be recreated.

Professor Wood commented that difficulties may arise if legal forms of practice were allowed to operate unchecked within the psychiatric system, and especially through the work of the mental health review tribunals. Although he regarded this as a danger which had not fully materialized, he was concerned that the representation of patients before the tribunals could become inappropriately adversarial. This theme linked directly to a more detailed discussion of the workings of the tribunal system.

Practical issues confronting the mental health review tribunals

Professor Wood suggested that the provision of annual reviews for all restricted patients may not be ideal, in so far as they might raise false hopes for patients whose crimes would have carried a very lengthy prison sentence without a clinical diagnosis. Further, with the tribunals now having responsibility for discharge, the whole hearing turned explicitly on this issue, and the old 'sham', whereby the tribunals made an effort to sympathetically appraise the patient's progress, before writing to the Home Office who made the decision could no longer operate. These hearings early in a patient's period of detention were now quite obviously pointless. Thus, despite the important work of MIND in securing these rights for patients, unfortunate consequences had ensued. Indeed, patients might feel that, with release depending largely upon the good nature of those listening, reviews were hardly a legal process at all.

However, it was suggested that the independence of the review tribunals from the Home Office was to be valued, in that it required the Home Office to explain its position with respect to the patient. Further, a number of contributors suggested that patients valued the annual reviews. Even if patients realized that their chances of release were slim, they valued the independence of the review as being quite separate from the hospital providing treatment. In particular, it was suggested that patients valued the hearings because they gave them a chance to gain information about the medical view of their progress, and to sit down with the doctors and discover what was happening to them. In this sense, the hearings might be regarded as having an important therapeutic function. It was argued that avoiding tribunals for those diagnosed as psychopathic would constitute a cynical acceptance of the incarceration and punishment of individuals in hospital.

Others spoke in support of Professor Wood's concerns. The findings of the Carlisle Committee concerning parole provisions for prisoners were referred to, where it was suggested that a similar picture emerged, with prisoners becoming bitter about being pressured by relatives and others to go through pointless parole hearings. One contributor felt that organizations representing patients actually ended up complying with the system; raising the hopes of patients when it was certain that the medical and Home Office view was unassailable. However, there was still a need for independent scrutiny of restriction orders.

One particularly marked problem discussed was that of securing places for patients ready for discharge from the special hospitals, with many having to wait for unacceptable periods of time for a suitable placement to be negotiated. It was suggested that this could be remedied by linking budgets to each patient rather than allocating them to institutions. With specific allocations of money following each patient round the sytem, there would be a financial incentive to take them on. The point was made that patients might enjoy specific rights of redress concerning the application and continuance of orders under the Mental Health Acts, but that they lacked general remedies with respect to health authorities and social services departments who fail to provide the services they require; some form of right to treatment legislation might be required.

It was pointed out by one contributor that the Mental Health Act Commission had only the limited remit of looking after the interests of detained patients. Also of concern were the possibility of the *de facto* detention of informal patients and the problems faced by the mentally disordered offender within the prison system. It was suggested that the Prisons Inspectorate was not equipped to look after the mentally disordered, while the Boards of Visitors were too identified with the authorities and lacked medical input. There was thus a case for the remit of the Mental Health Act Commission to be extended. In addition, the

Commission should be less obsessed with 'the visit', and should act as a prompter of research and accumulator and dissimulator of information (it has some data on psychosurgery).

Notes

1. A much publicized case, that of Beverley Lewis, reported on 31 October 1989 led to the call for the recasting of compulsory guardianship powers so as to permit social workers to protect a mentally impaired, blind and deaf young woman by seeking a guardianship order under the Mental Health Act 1983. This Act appears to give such powers but defines mental impairment as involving being 'abnormally aggressive or seriously irresponsible' – s.1(2). It seems social workers felt the law would not see complete inability to look after oneself as 'seriously irresponsible'. If that is right, which may be doubted, the statute omits the most obvious need for guardianship; a belated discovery indeed.
2. Basically the Mental Health Act 1983 and the Mental Health Tribunal Rules 1983.
3. The adversarial approach is seen in a recent book by Cavidino which makes the suggestion that the authorized social worker, considering a compulsory admission, should act as arbiter between doctor and patient, surely a dangerous confusion of functions (Cavadino, 1989).
4. It is, for example, possible to recall occasions where a responsible medical officer has told a mental health review tribunal that if the patient is discharged he will not undertake the patient's care again.
5. Mental Health Act 1983 s.1(2) '. . . Mental illness, arrested or incomplete development of mind, psychopathic disorder and any other disorder or disability of mind . . .'; a definition made very wide by the last clause.
6. A patient has spent the last seven years in Rampton on the transfer list.
7. In the case of Secretary of State for the Home Department v Mental Health Review Tribunal for Mersey Regional Health Authority (1986) I WLR 1170. It was emphasized that the tribunal powers set out in s.72 of the Mental Health Act 1983 used the word 'discharge' which did not cover compulsory transfer to another hospital.
8. R v Kaye (1988) *The Times*, 25 May. The Court of Appeal supported the approval by the Divisional Court of the tribunal's action. It could be argued that what should be discharged by the tribunal is the order, not the patient, but the Act prevents this logical approach by speaking of the discharge of the patient.
9. R v Mersey Mental Health Review Tribunal Ex p Dillon, 19 March 1986.
10. Mental Health Act 1983, s.145.
11. R v The Nottingham Mental Health Review Tribunal Ex p Secretary of State for the Home Department (Thomas) and R v Trent Mental Health Review Tribunal Ex p Secretary of State for the Home Department, 15 September 1988.
12. Ex p Waldron (1985) 3 WLR 1090.
13. A recent survey is to be found in Bean 1986. Although it has many proposals for reform, it cannot be said that these, even if all accepted, would amount to major reconstruction. Jill Peay's empirical research on the work of the mental health review tribunals has appeared as an important book (Peay, 1989). The result of her proposals is also likely to be considerable reform rather than fundamental restructuring.

4

A criminological perspective – the influence of fashion and theory on practice and disposal: life chances in the criminological tombola

J. PEAY[1]

The aim of my paper is to take King's (1981) theoretical models of the criminal justice system and impose on them the major changes of the last 40 years in the ways of dealing with mentally disordered offenders. The paper's rationale is that adequately to provide for the future requires an understanding of the costs and benefits of tried and tired methods. Along the route I plan to examine: (i) whether there is any sufficient justification for dealing with mentally disordered offenders as a special and isolated group; (ii) if not, whether categorization as a 'mentally disordered offender' constitutes a form of unmerited negative or positive discrimination; and (iii) how developments in the penal and therapeutic systems have brought them closer together ideologically, without any prerequisite examination of whether it is necessary to have two different systems co-existing. Two themes recur throughout the critique. First, the theoretical basis for separation is overly rigid, relying as it does upon false and outmoded dichotomies. Secondly, at a practical level, the existence of parallel systems is unsound. The paper, therefore, is intentionally provocative, its aim being to challenge the assumptions behind the status quo, whilst tentatively advancing an alternative pluralist model.

I need to stress from the outset that I will not principally be dealing with the clear-cut ends of the illness-offending or mad-bad spectrum, but with those who fall in the 'muddied central arena' or the 'perpetual twilight' (re *Golden Chemical Products Ltd*, 1976) where the decision might go either way. Just as that tiny minority of the patently insane do not merit punishment, I do not intend to agonize over the 'disposal' of the tiny proportion of the wilful, calculated and cruel.

The perspective I've been asked to adopt is that of a criminologist and here I plan to draw on the Sutherland and Cressey definition of criminology (quoted in Prins, 1982) as being that 'body of knowledge regarding crime as a social phenomenon. It includes within its scope the processes of making laws, and of reacting towards the breaking of laws' (p. 10). Three main divisions of criminology are recognized: (i) the sociology of law; (ii) the study of the causes of crime; and (iii) penology – the control and treatment of crime. It is my view that these areas are not wholly distinct, interacting as they do with one another. My paper ranges promiscuously across all three.

Theoretical models of criminal justice

Of King's (1981) six theoretical, if recognizably artificial, models of the criminal justice system this paper will focus on three; namely, crime control, due process and the medical model. These are not regarded as explanatory models, but rather as devices to illustrate the themes which have been dominant in much of the recent literature on mentally disordered offenders. Nor should any of these models be regarded as operating in a vacuum. Notably, the three models have not been applied even handedly to the so-called 'normal' offender and the disordered offender; their presentation here is a caricature of King's thorough analysis.

Packer (1969) has argued that the criminal justice system could be seen as a conflict between two competing value systems, namely crime control (which I will identify as giving primacy to societal or 'greater good' interests) and due process (where the emphasis is on the individual's best interests/needs).

In the crime control model the primary object is the repression of criminal conduct through punishment, either by deterring others or by deterring the specific offender from re-offending.

The quantity of punishment is moderated by the harm caused and the offender's blameworthiness, thereby sustaining the model's moral overtones. There is a necessary assumption that people are fully responsible for their behaviour.[2] Co-existing with notions of morality are utilitarian objectives, for crime control adopts the view that the welfare of the greatest number is all important: inflicting suffering on an individual is a permissible evil provided sufficient benefits accrue to the rest of the population. In this sense, rules of procedure and evidence are obstacles to conviction; a high conviction rate rather than just convictions are paramount.

In stark contrast due process promotes as its social function justice and fairness. The model emphasizes the possibility of error particularly in informal and pre-adjudicative activities. In order to avoid unjust punishment, the model insists upon procedural safeguards and adherence to formal rules and adversary processes. 'Quality control' along the route is therefore all important (Packer, 1969). Notably, the model emphasizes primacy of the individual's interests where conflict exists between individual and state, even if this reduces the state's effectiveness in controlling crime.

A third approach relates to rehabilitation and the medical model. Like the crime control model, crimes are primarily a reason for social intervention. Yet, in contrast, free-will is perceived as an illusion. As behaviour is a product of events beyond people's control, its central imperative entails meeting offenders' needs and thereby permitting them greater control over future behaviour (logically a problematic concept in itself). At its crudest, the role of the court is as a diagnostician: all are in need of 'treatment' – the question concerns appropriate allocation, which requires relevant information, the diagnosis of the causes of anti-social acts and proposing appropriate courses of treatment. However, the model does require the courts to be receptive to the responses of individuals to the 'treatment' allocated; the rationale is not to treat like cases alike, but to discover what works. The model's focus on effectiveness and the reduction of future offending provides an overlap with crime control, but it is individualized, giving the model some superficial similarities with due process (i.e. what is in the individual's interests because, ultimately, this is the most effective route to serving societal interests). Since this therapeutic assessment makes an individual's rights of secondary importance, the objective of the reduction of offending is likely to be achieved at some cost to the competing due process model; for example, treatment without consent. Yet on the positive side, therapeutic endeavours and due process may pull in the same direction; for example, the disclosure of reports to patients.

All three models have been criticized (e.g. McBarnet, 1981) with the medical model being subject to the greatest criticism; comprehensively discredited as 'theoretically faulty, systematically discriminatory in application, and inconsistent with some of our most basic concepts of justice' (American Friends Service Committee, 1971: p. 21) and of no proven reformative value (Croft, 1978). Yet, as is evident below, it remains the predominant model, admittedly now tempered by greater due process considerations, for the mentally disordered offender.

Developments in the management of mentally disordered offenders in the criminal justice system

The criminal justice system is thus subject to conflicting pressures deriving from societal and individual interests. They find various expression in the three models above. How then have these models manifested themselves in relation to the mentally disordered offender in the last 40 years?

Stage 1: (Pre Mental Health Act 1959/Homicide Act 1957)

Pre-conviction offenders were divided into the 'mad' and 'bad' via the insanity defence (not guilty by reason of insanity). This approach was dominated by the crime control model. Where offenders were not responsible, is was considered inappropriate to convict or punish, their fate being detention (and treatment) at Her Majesty's pleasure at a secure psychiatric hospital.[3] Offenders were, in essence, divided into the punishable and the non-punishable. Mental disorder was relevant for other offenders only to mitigate punishment, not fundamentally to alter its quality.

The problems with this model are:

(*a*) The divisions between punishment and treatment are not clearly demarcated: professional and recipient perceptions of needs may not be at one; treatment in the context of indefinite detention may feel like punishment; punishment may in itself be a form of 'treatment' (if re-offending does not occur). Thus, although not wishing to dissent from the ancient and humane principle that the mentally ill should be neither convicted nor punished (Dell, 1983) it might be asserted that the reality of then existent arrangements paid lip service in open court to that principle, whilst the subjective reality permitted both the stigma of 'conviction' (not guilty by reason of insanity) and the experience of prolonged confinement.

(*b*) Where avoidance of conviction depends upon legal (moderated by medical) assessments of responsibility, what are the logical limits to the division into punishable and non-punishable as our understanding of human behaviour becomes more sophisticated? As Griew

(1984) asserts, responsibility is a muddying word as it conflates notions of capacity and liability. If it were to be proven, for example, that an abnormally low white blood cell count affected the individual's ability to understand the consequences of his or her actions where would that leave the insanity defence?

(c) Allocation may have been subject to due process in court, but subsequent release was not – being subject to executive/medical discretion.

(d) Most importantly, the arrangements allow for the uncomfortable probability that we end up punishing the mentally ill (as the vast majority of offenders with mental disorders made no use of the insanity defence); and, given that the prison system is so dehumanizing, punishment becomes both unjustifiably severe and patently ineffective for the mentally disordered. Almost any alternative looks more attractive.

Thus, too much of the debate was fruitlessly locked into questions such as 'Is he responsible?', 'What is the precise relationship between crime and disorder and therefore can he be punished?' Arguably, the subsequent shift in the debate to the utilitarian approach which allowed symbolic convictions followed by 'What's best in the interests of the individual with mental disorder at the point of sentence?' resulted in an exponential expansion of the categories of offender to whom we were preparing to allow entry to the medical model.

Stage 2 (Post 1959/1983 Mental Health Acts and the 1957 Homicide Act)

This entailed a drift from the crime control moral perspective looking at questions of responsibility, to the crime control utilitarian approach, resulting in an overlap with the medical model. It accepted that reality required pragmatism; a range of resources existed and the real question concerned matching them to individuals' needs, tempered by due process.

Offenders were divided into the punishable and the treatable. For the latter group, the opportunity to punish (DHSS *et al.*, 1978) or rather to punish overtly, was foregone. There was no substantial separation prior to conviction (although the insanity defence is retained) as responsibility is no longer the key issue at trial. Separation occurs at sentence into the more realistic 'partly mad and partly bad' (Verdun-Jones, 1989).

The problems with this model are:

(*a*) Once the division is made, the system slips back into its inflexible mould. For the mentally disordered, it is a 'one-way street'; even normal offenders are only entitled to the benefits of treatment via transfer in the context of the possibility of being returned to a penal environment.

(*b*) For the punishable, sentencing is primarily retributive within the crime control model. Its limitations are well documented, with its advantages being primarily the fixed and, arguably, reduced length of detention.

(*c*) For the 'treatable', effectiveness is judged by medical criteria. If the patient fails these, then the consequences may be a longer and uncertain period in hospital. Indeed, length of stay may be prolonged on the grounds of attributed dangerousness (even though this is not a legitimate criterion). Finally, where there is no effective treatment available, the patient may be detained on the grounds of the seriousness of offence – resulting in intervention constituting covert preventive indefinite detention as Dell and Robertson (1988) showed for psychopaths.

(*d*) Critically, this second stage does not, in practice, wholly avoid the debate about responsibility. For the mentally disordered, at the point of release the relationship between crime and disorder re-emerges, despite its official irrelevance (Peay, 1989) and in spite of the system of procedural safeguards enjoyed by the mentally disordered offender/patient. Arguments about the probability of the patient re-offending if released abound, even where the basis for continued confinement is legally justifiable only where the individual continues to suffer from a mental disorder which warrants detention in hospital for medical treatment. Arguably, the influence of the crime control model has just been shifted through the criminal justice system. To do away with it completely would require rigid adherence to the inappropriateness of looking at 'dangerousness' in release criteria.

Given English law's historical interest in remedies, that is a pragmatic concern with outcomes, which in turn give rights (as illustrated by the introduction of the mental health review tribunal system), it might be argued that the law relating to mentally disordered offenders has had a remedial basis, but not a principled approach. Adopting remedies for the mentally disordered drove them down the medical model route, with its anticipation of future harm, whereas remedies for normal offenders resulted in proportionality in punishment, with its focus on the assessment of present and past behaviour. Yet, this may be a false and discriminatory dichotomy. Has the development of two parallel systems for normal and abnormal offenders resulted in unjustifiable consequences in terms of their life chances?

Should we recognize 'the mentally disordered offender' as an isolated category?

In much the same way that we are only just beginning to accept that criminals and victims are not separate categories – most offenders have been victims, many victims have been offenders (Jones & Young, 1989) – I would argue that it is better to speak of offenders with mental disorders and mentally disordered people who commit crimes, or even people who have committed crimes and experience mental disorder, rather than the global 'mentally disordered offender'. Many offenders will, in mitigation, point to their mental state, without raising it as an explicit defence. Moreover, given the incidence of psychiatric disorder in the prison population, there are clearly many offenders with mental disorders in prisons rather than in hospital (Home Office, 1978b, 1987b). In health care terms, their numbers are high. Yet, why should only those in hospital be singled out for special measures and special help? And why only those with a mental disability of sufficient severity arising at a particular time and in a particular context; once the obsessive focus on responsibility has gone why should we not equally single out as special those with, for example, physical disabilities?

Moreover, the concept of the mentally disordered offender is itself problematic (Hollin, 1989); the inferential leap required to establish that the presence of a disordered mind has caused the offending behaviour is sufficiently wide to place the burden on those who wish to assert the truth of the proposition. For the majority where the two classifications of mental disorder and offender co-exist, there can be no proven causal connection, and for those who become ill after the commission of their crimes and before sentence the possibility that they might be classified as a mentally disordered offender is peculiarly inappropriate.

Abnormal behaviour *per se* cannot be a legitimate criterion given that what is 'abnormal' is culturally and legally defined: at times of war, for example, those who are singled out as meriting special intervention are those who are unable to kill.

Even where the accused's abnormal state of mind is a legitimate issue at trial, the consequences of raising the spectre of 'mental disorder bordering on insanity' are, for the accused and the legal system's sense of balance, horrendous. Suddenly, the focus is no longer on what the accused is alleged to have done, but rather on who (or even 'what') he is. All manner of inconsistencies emerge and are tolerated by the courts: defendants pleading to offences they have not committed in order to avoid the consequences of a finding of not guilty by reason of insanity (*Quick; Sullivan; Clarke*); bizarre decisions which argue that the diabetic who offends during a hypoglycaemic attack should be eligible to walk entirely free from the court (*Quick*), whilst he who offends during a hyperglycaemic episode risks indefinite detention in a maximum security hospital (*Hennessy*); and the failure of the courts to find an effective means to achieve 'intervention' in the life of a man who admits to repeatedly raping and kicking a woman who is a stranger to him (*Ratahi*). Arguably then, the law's conceptual shift before conviction not only discriminates against the offender with a mental disorder, but in some circumstances discriminates unjustifiably in his favour and thereby also seriously disadvantages society as a whole.

Setting on one side the pre-conviction inconsistencies, what sense can be made of the sentencing stage? For both 'mentally disordered' offenders and some 'normal' offenders the focus is individualized with the form of intervention being designed to fit the offender (but within limits for the normal offender and with their consent normally being a prerequisite for an individualized sentence, e.g. probation). But, there is a catalogue of research to show that decision-makers are cognitively ill-equipped to make complex decisions (Konecni *et al.*, 1980) and that only one or two factors have a remarkable influence on disposal. Moreover, when faced with expert evidence relating to the offender's treatment needs, the arbitrariness of decisions is heightened. Genuine exchange of discourses may not be possible; empirical research has illustrated that the prevailing domain holds sway – so that in legal settings the medical approach takes a back seat (Chiswick, 1985) with the reverse in medical settings (Peay, 1989). Each may draw on the resources of alternative arguments to support predetermined outcomes (Denning in *Bratty* and see Menzies' (1987) study of forensic practitioners[4]). Ultimately, the medicalization of due process (courts following medical recommendations) is both limited and arguably inappropriate because it replaces legal definitions of patients' rights with doctors' definitions of patients' needs. Access to hospital places is medically determined; the courts can only overrule a medical recommendation to order punishment (as occurred in *Gunnell* and *Castro*), yet the courts cannot order treatment, even where the due process approach suggests that is the right course, if a bed is not made available in an appropriate hospital (*Mental Health Act* 1983 s.37 [4]).

In essence, my argument is that the whole is less than the sum of the parts; in their present form the co-existence of medical and penal approaches disadvantages both, but peculiarly disadvantages the 'mentally disordered offender'. From the beginning to the end of the process, as the conjunction of Teplin and Pruett's (1992) study and Parker (1980) shows, the mentally disordered on the streets are more likely to be arrested and charged for similar offences than their normal peers (in order to meet treatment needs) whilst ultimately mentally disordered offenders may be kept longer in therapeutic settings (on protective grounds). Flexibility in the theoretical justifications employed, disadvantages the disordered offender without the necessary spin-off in concomitant safeguards.

Thus, given both vagaries in the allocation of individuals to the 'mentally disordered' group and the limitations of intervention thereafter, I would argue that there is no sufficient justification for treating them as an isolated group.

The advantages and disadvantages of parallel systems

At this stage Potas' (1982) assertion that it is in the name of rehabilitation that the greatest threats are posed to individual rights and liberties bears repetition. Having parallel systems will result in some benefiting and some suffering from their co-existence. Indeed, perhaps the appearance of better treatment disguises from a patient perspective a more punitive but equally ineffective approach. And from the normal offender's perspective it might be argued that as due process entails positive discrimination for the mentally disordered, this is only achieved at the resource expense of those within the penal system. Not only is there less cake but the moral imperative for sharing it equally is less pressing once it can be argued that those in greater need – the mentally disordered offenders – should have the bigger slice. Thus, normal offenders may receive even less 'treatment'. Should not all offenders be given equal opportunity of access to 'benefits'?

Clearly, the mentally disordered serious offender (serious offence, not serious disorder, see *R v Birch*) risks double jeopardy. Indefinite detention is superseded by delayed release on grounds of dangerousness.

Equally, the discretionary life sentenced prisoner may find his mental disorder serves to increase (not decrease) the severity of punishment (Verdun-Jones, 1989). Dangerousness is overly subject to medical expertise and that may disproportionately and unfairly influence the court's sentencing strategy.

Thus, the disadvantages in life chances underline the argument for doing away with 'mentally disordered offenders' as an isolated group, or, if the category is to be retained, ensuring that its application is carefully constrained or its consequences moderated.

Arguably a very small group may remain in whom responsibility is negated (Taylor, 1985). Some form of insanity defence would need to be retained. But why not along the lines proposed by the Butler Committee (Home Office/DHSS, 1975) which would have as great an impact on the evidential aspects of the trial process, leaving the traditional burden on the prosecution, in order to establish the defence of 'not guilty on evidence of mental disorder'? Such a proposal already has authoritative support (Dell, 1983; Griew, 1984) and sections of the Draft Criminal Code seek to implement the Butler recommendations in a modified form.[5] Yet, why not also enhance the changes brought about by the *Mental Health Act* 1983 which provide review by tribunal for those detained under s.5 of the *Criminal Procedure (Insanity) Act* 1964?[6] Why not reinforce the burden on the detaining authority by specifying that they have to satisfy the tribunal beyond reasonable doubt that further detention is required? And why not impart to the courts a complete sentencing discretion where a finding of 'no sufficient *mens rea* by reason of mental disorder' occurs? Such an approach may enhance the attractiveness of running the defence and thereby extend its ambit to the hopeless and helpless in cases where prosecution cannot be avoided because of the seriousness of the alleged offence.

The similarities and dissimilarities of the parallel systems

A case can be made for suggesting that recent developments in the penal and therapeutic methods of control of offenders have resulted in a growing similarity, rather than dissimilarity, between the two. Calls for treatment in prison of, for example, sex offenders and the possible expansion of therapeutic approaches as exemplified by Grendon Underwood Prison are likely to result in a blurring of the boundaries.

Parallel developments in the field of civil commitment, arising out of a recognition that 'mental health' legislation is discriminatory, have included the progressive return to patients of their civil rights. Equally, in the penal setting there have been calls for the normalization of prison medical services (King & Morgan, 1980; Home Office, 1990*b*).

Similarly, the 'long leash' approach – the clarion call of the movement for community treatment orders for the mentally disordered – has become fashionable in the face of fierce opposition (Fennell, 1992). This has many similarities both in respect of the theoretical debate associated with parole and in its practical arrangements.[7] Moreover, crime control advocates have regularly pointed to the merits of control in the community as a means of reducing offending.

Yet the system of release is perhaps the most telling area. Shifting discretion to the decision to release causes as many difficulties in respect of due process for those in penal institutions as in psychiatric settings. Utilitarian objectives, with their reliance on prediction, become paramount. But trading off societal interests in the prevention of further offending and individual interests (which were after all the justification for going down this route in the first instance) is never likely to be easy. The requisite due process safeguards are an accepted part of discharge for mentally disordered offenders in treatment setting (*Tribunals & Inquiries Act* 1958); patients enjoy the advantages of mental health review tribunals with all the benefits they bring in terms of disclosure of information, etc. Increasingly they have been called for in penal settings.[8] However, although natural justice is now applicable to Boards of Visitors and may become so for Governors' hearings (Wade, 1988) there is, as yet, no genuine comparability between the procedural safeguards enjoyed by patients and those of prisoners where their basic rights and welfare are arguably being overlooked.

Clearly, there is support for revising the system of parole hearings to ensure more judicial style hearings with reasons being given, if not representation (Home Office, 1988*a*). Yet the fundamental dissimilarity remains. For the normal offender not on a life sentence, imprisonment means the prospect of certain release combined with the possibility of parole, whilst patients on restriction orders have the prospect of prolonged, indefinite detention combined with the on-going possibility of release occurring earlier in their period of confinement.[9] Does 'treatment' make this a price worth paying? Is it one that can be justified? Has what has been held out in theory as positive discrimination been negative discrimination in practice?

Moreover, research has demonstrated that even with the system of procedural safeguards for patients, crime control tends to creep in by the back door. And the fact that this does not receive official condemnation is an index of the preparedness to treat the mentally disordered by a different yardstick; name the rules of the game and then use and abuse them. Indeed, the recent Consultation Document *Offenders Suffering from Psychopathic Disorder* (Home Office, 1986*a*) was arguably an expedient measure aimed at the preventative detention of this group (Peay, 1988). The diagnosis, therefore, would have served, not as a basis to classify them for their benefit, but to differentiate to their detriment. Thus, have we arguably spent too long thinking of mentally disordered offenders as falling into discrete diagnostic categories which start out as justifying their special treatment but end up justifying their special punishment? That is the risk, as has materialized in the defects addressed here, which discrete classification and parallel systems face.

Are these unfairnesses in life chances either theoretically justifiable or practically efficacious? The present system has been shown to be deficient in a number of respects. Amongst these are that the system is reliant on medical discretion; it fails to identify and deal with all offenders with mental disorders; it dissuades those who might benefit from treatment from exposing themselves to it and encourages them to choose the seemingly preferable certainty of (inappropriate) conviction; it fails to safeguard 'rights' to release; it resorts to indefinite and preventative detention; it uses and abuses labels as means to ends; and it fails to give sentencers sufficient discretion to do justice to the objectives of prosecution. In this context, what alternatives propose themselves?

Punish, treat, help: isolate or combine?

It would, of course, be possible to recommend a series of improvements to the existing systems for dealing with offenders who experience mental disorder, and those who do not, as a way of resolving the deficiencies, disparities and discriminatory aspects of the arrangements reviewed above. However, my purpose here has not been merely to advocate a multitude of tinkerings in order to edge towards an ideal (and, some may argue, idealized) system. Rather, my aim has been to throw down a challenge to those who would wish to support the *status quo* by examining whether the fundamentals of the present system can be justified. In this spirit, my conclusions are tentative and deliberately provocative. In essence, they strive to sketch the possibilities of a more thorough review of the fundamentals of both theory and practice.

Although the arguments about why a just deserts/proportionality approach would be inappropriate for mentally disordered offenders have been well rehearsed (DHSS *et al.*, 1978) they remain valid only in so far as one accepts the premise that offenders with mental disorders should be treated as an isolated group.[10]

If one starts from the assumption that the system has been outcome driven (i.e. that it is repugnant to inflict the reality of punishment on the mentally ill and appealing to offer them the fantasy of treatment) then there is a need to examine the labels more closely. This process has resulted in an assessment that the labels may be discriminatory in themselves. For example, Walker & McCabe's (1973) incisive assertion in respect of psychopathic disorder that the law has offered the psychiatrist a ready-made label which will help him to get his patient through 'the customs barrier of the courts' (p. 235) leaves open the consequences for the offender. Whether these consequences are perceived as positive or negative may depend not only on what treatment is available, but for how long one has to experience it. Moreover, the reality for those with mental disorders is that crime control, despite its seeming rejection at the public sentencing stage, creeps in again at the back door of release. It is the reality and not the rhetoric which must be confronted. The individual's perspective and the context in which it is formed may be more important than the immediate label 'punishment' or 'treatment'. It is then the real consequences of the labels which are all important, not whether the court is seen to keep its hands clean by not punishing the mentally disordered (or not providing the advantages of treatment to the punishable). Indeed, punishment and treatment are labels and may make no long-term difference (depending on the perspective adopted: time in detention, effectiveness, etc.). It is not whether the labels themselves stick and influence chances in the long-term, but how in the short-term they have social consequences in respect of allocation.

An alternative approach therefore may be to question whether perhaps all should be treated equally (due process model) or that all may be treatable (the humanitarian face of the medical model) or that all are equally punishable. If it is only the barbaric aspects of our present system of imprisonment which makes this last alternative anathema, this would seem a justification for providing more humane containment, with due process review procedures and 'treatment' opportunities (in the guise of 'help' [Bottoms & McWilliams, 1979]) in a penal setting at the offender's request and with his consent. If the true demand for classification is for allocation purposes, then if we do away with distinctions in allocation at the court stage we also do away with the need for labels. The sole question of 'Can he be punished?' is replaced by a number of key issues including 'Will he have access to treatment?'

In essence, one pluralist model is being proposed because the three 'options' above, although labelled differently, could in practice be different aspects of the same system. Support for this kind of rationale within our interventionist practices may be seen in the work of Dell and Robertson (1988), who argue for greater interchange between prison and hospital whilst retaining fixed sentences for the psychopathically disordered. Similiarly, Richardson (1988) argues for an extension of due process safeguards throughout the periods of disposal and treatment for mentally disordered offenders and lifers. Genders & Player (1989) argue on the basis of research at Grendon Prison that it is not possible under the present methods of assessment to determine who will benefit from a stay at the prison and that those who palpably do benefit are not necessarily those predicted as most likely to do so. Dickens (1985), argues that dangerousness should be a legal status and subject to due process; and my own research shows that procedural safeguards in their present form are insufficient in scope and ineffective in practice when countering the powerful 'crime control' arguments. If the partly mad can be partly bad and thereby partly punishable, why can't the partly bad benefit from the nature and quality of the services offered to the partly mad? This is, of course, not to assert that all would be treated alike, but merely to recognize that the existing arrangements are too inflexible and deny access to opportunities on the basis of a theoretical separation which cannot be sustained.

The approach which is being advocated would necessitate re-examining each of the different stages of pre-conviction, conviction, allocation, confinement, release and reintegration. While permitting movement between the range of interventions available, the model would be equally flexible in the theoretical emphases adopted at each stage, but consistent within stages. So, for example, responsibility might constitute the basis for conviction, but the nature of an offender's confinement might be determined by the therapeutic criterion of treatability in combination with his or her consent, while release would be governed by the severity of the offence actually committed and not according to medical criteria. Hollin (1989) citing Washbrook (1981: p. 127) notes 'More and more the psychiatric hospital must move towards the hospital for physical illness and likewise there must be a tendency to push prisons towards the psychiatric hospital model'. Equally, there are aspects of our penal arrangements, with their emphasis on justice and fairness, which therapeutic systems should seek to mirror. This paper is not a plea for the re-adoption of the medical model *per se*, but rather a recognition that the time is well past when there should be a balancing of the peculiar merits of each model to provide one cohesive system capable of dealing with the particular conditions of all, rather than our present attempt to divide the goods according to an artificially rigid and unworkable understanding of criminal behaviour, mental disorder and their relationship. Pluralism works, OK?

Discussion

Much of the discussion was pitched at a general level, in keeping with both Dr Peay's paper and her presentation. Contributions focused on the legal implications of a psychiatric diagnosis for the accused and the convicted, and on the complexities of the modern medico-legal system. There was a more concrete discussion concerning diversion of the mentally disordered from prosecution, both by the police and the Crown Prosecution Service.

Legal and clinical implications of a psychiatric diagnosis

In discussion, the central question addressed by Dr Peay in her paper was raised again; is it a good fate for an offender to be diagnosed as mentally disordered? Further, is it best to be placed in a specialist institution such as a special hospital or a regional secure unit where appropriate, or is the patient better off in a well-run long-term general psychiatric hospital? Dr Peay drew a distinction between the patient's short-term and long-term fate. Those who had been in prison and hospital preferred hospital, but a long-term psychiatric placement may not be advantageous. With respect to the special hospitals, one contributor clarified the patients' usual response at Broadmoor Hospital; they liked the physical aspects of the hospital, but not the indeterminacy of their detention. Thus, the offender was not deemed by the contributors to suffer through a psychiatric diagnosis in terms of the setting of their detention, but its duration, and particularly its indeterminacy.

A number of changes in the situation of offenders diagnosed as mentally disordered were noted. In general, it was suggested that, in the past, people placed in psychiatric hospitals had not been thought responsible for their actions, but that this was no longer necessarily the case. With respect to transfers from prison, it was suggested that 'psychopaths' who were very disturbed, but who showed no signs of psychosis might not, in practice, be transferred to hospital. Although they could be defined as mentally disordered on the basis of their psychopathy, it was argued that this procedure was not tight enough, and that it was difficult to transfer such individuals to a secure hospital. These comments applied to the situation in England and Wales. In Scotland, the criteria for a diagnosis and placement on the basis of psychopathy existed, although the legal category of psychopathic disorder was not included in the equivalent Scottish mental health legislation. In Northern Ireland, a diagnosis of personality disorder is insufficient for the purposes of detention.

Non-prosecution: the 'public interest' option

There was considerable discussion about mechanisms by which mentally disordered offenders might be diverted from the criminal justice system altogether. It was noted that there might be considerable regional disparities in the response of police officers to the mentally disordered. The police had great discretion in the treatment of individuals, particularly those arrested for minor offences. The use of s.136 of the *Mental Health Act* 1983 to detain an apparently disordered individual in a place of safety varied considerably.

There was a lengthy discussion concerning the option of non-prosecution where prosecution was deemed not to be in the 'public interest'. It was suggested that this might lead to civil prosecutions in which the mentally disordered had little protection. Dr Peay argued that, on practical grounds, the Crown Prosecution Service should always be reluctant to prosecute the mentally disordered because of the difficulty of obtaining a conviction. In any event, she suggested, there were safeguards for patients facing civil actions. However, she was concerned that the 'public interest' criterion was not being used with any rigour; there was no sticking to the philosophy or the text of the Crown Prosecution Service Code of Practice. In particular, at present, all information that came to the CPS was furnished by the police and tended to be geared towards prosecution. (Graham Smith's chapter describes a Public Interest Case Assessment project designed to encourage the CPS to avoid prosecution of the mentally disordered where possible.) It was suggested that, if rapid alternatives to prosecution existed, the CPS would use them, but they were at present likely to prosecute the violent mentally disordered offender in order to protect the public.

The question of the desirability of testing the guilt or innocence of the mentally disordered was raised. One contributor, referring to the mentally handicapped, suggested that sometimes it was necessary to encourage a prosecution so that the facts were tested, although a trial could be a great ordeal for the accused. However, it was pointed out that a trial does not necessarily take the case further forward in this respect. One particularly worrying possibility is that the prosecution is used as a means of placing a hospital patient in prison 'to make him responsible for his actions'.

Rigidity and flexibility in a complex system of provision

It was argued that a whole range of decision-making points existed where the needs of the mentally disordered should be considered within the criminal justice system. Not only were too many mentally disordered individuals prosecuted, but too many were remanded in custody and too many were sentenced. In order to avoid this, it was suggested that the health care system needed to be more efficient and rapid in response. In particular, the delay in providing reports was highlighted.

It was argued that some mechanism needed to be found to ensure that, in the case of those offenders diagnosed as mentally disordered, the length of detention remained based on the gravity of the offence. Dr Peay repeated her call for an end to the hospital order whilst retaining the availability of hospital or hospital-like facilities for all who needed them in the criminal justice system.

Notes

1. I am greatly indebted to both Andrew Ashworth and Andrew Halpin for their comments on earlier drafts of this paper. Neither would necessarily wish to be associated with my conclusions, but both have been influential in formulating and clarifying my thinking.
2. Or where self-control is lost, that there was an earlier conscious choice made to risk its loss, for example through intoxication.
3. The popular American alternative being guilty but mentally ill. Treatment is still recognized as being the most appropriate action. The verdict is accepted as nothing more than a label whose precise nature may affect juries' willingness to apply it. In the long-term, the label merely signifies that punishment *per se* is inappropriate.

4. Menzies (1987) noted that 'the legalistic ecology of (the assessment unit) was associated with a wholesale abandonment of traditional psychiatric orientations, and with an emphasis instead upon conceptions of responsibility, correctionalism and penality'. Moreover, Menzies asserted that the psychiatric assessments provided 'an apparent medical framework for the allocation of penal measures'.
5. See, for example, clauses 33–34 of the Draft Criminal Code (Law Commission, 1989).
6. The *Criminal Procedure (Insanity) Act* 1964 has now been replaced by the *Criminal Procedure (Insanity and Unfitness to Plead) Act* 1991, which came into force on 1 January 1992, and which introduces a flexible range of disposals.
7. And all the overtones of failing to ensure the provision of adequate community care and deal with the real causes of mental disorder; just as parole continues to place responsibility on the individual rather than looking at the social and economic factors which contribute to crime.
8. See the discussion of the Prior Report on prison disciplinary hearings (Home Office, 1985) and the Government's White Paper (Home Office, 1986*b*) followed by their ultimate rejection of both the need to split the Boards of Visitors' adjudicative and watchdog roles and substantive procedural safeguards (McKittrick, 1987). However, more recently the report of the Woolf Inquiry has recommended that standards of justice within prisons should be improved and that Boards of Visitors should be relieved of their adjudicatory role (Home Office, 1991).
9. For the position in respect of life sentenced prisoners see the recommendations of the House of Lords Select Committee on Murder and Life Imprisonment (October 1989) previewed in Windlesham (1989).
10. Even though the offender's attributed responsibility for his actions is no longer the key issue, those found to be partially responsible (i.e. with verdicts of diminished responsibility) are variously treated: in the first instance as wholly responsible; subsequently as amongst the potentially treatable; whilst ultimately, as for all offender patients, the issue of responsibility may determine release.

Part III

Perspectives on future needs

5

The mentally abnormal offender in the era of community care

A. J. FOWLES[1]

Introduction

In the last two or three years popular attention has again been focused by the media on the fate of people discharged into the community from long-stay mental hospitals. Vivid images have been provided of the 'bag people' who were bused out of hospitals and were dropped off on successive street corners in New York City. Closer to home, people in contact with the courts can all provide anecdotal accounts of mentally ill people being imprisoned because no hospital place could be found for them. At the same time, official figures show an increase in the prison population together with a dramatic decrease in the population figures for mental hospitals. These two trends have been linked and some people have gone on to assume that we are witnessing a direct transfer of institutional populations.

The argument about the impact of community care seems to have been based more on speculation than hard data. An additional factor is the tendency to treat the policies which make up community care as if they were homogeneous and have been implemented synchronously across the health authorities of England and Wales. Detailed analysis of recent changes in institutional populations quickly reveals how little we really know about the people and processes involved.

The intention in this paper is to look in more detail at the changes in populations observed in prisons and mental hospitals – what has been called the 'transcarceration' hypothesis – and to look at the available evidence which has led to the argument that more mentally ill people are coming into contact with the criminal justice system. Brief references will be made to the American literature and data but as will be seen this tends to be of value only at a conceptual level.

The argument that changes in prison and mental hospital populations are linked is not new. Lionel Penrose put the idea forward in the 1930s but it has been given a new lease of life with the advent of de-institutionalization and community care. These two terms are often used interchangeably but, for our purposes, they are probably better treated as distinct terms especially as care in the community may be in short supply for those discharged from long-stay institutions. It is essential to interpret Penrose and some of those who have borrowed his ideas in the light of the remarks made by Paul Bowden in the following chapter. It is worth noting that contemporary changes in the size of institutional populations form part of a much longer historical span which cannot be dealt with here.

The 'transcarceration' hypothesis

When stated at its bluntest, the 'transcarceration' hypothesis is that as a result of the closure of mental hospitals there has been a shift of population to prisons. The idea is that one form of institutional setting has simply been substituted for another. The original intentions behind the closure of mental hospitals, greater personal freedom and a normal life in the community, have not been fulfilled. Former mental hospital patients have frequently been dumped in the community and many have been re-institutionalized but this time in the less appropriate surroundings of the prison. The failure of independent living may have been the result of inadequate, or non-existent, community facilities and/or dumping people in hostile communities unwilling to tolerate unconventional behaviour.

The idea of 'transcarceration' has been discussed recently in the United States where there has been a dramatic shift in institutional populations over the last two decades. Steadman *et al.* state that:

At the end of 1968, there were 39 000 patients in state mental hospitals and 168 000 inmates in state prisons. Within a decade, the hospital population fell 64% to 147 000 and the prison population rose 65% to 277 000.'

(Steadman *et al.* 1984: p. 475)

Not only did prison populations rise while state mental hospital populations fell, but the rate of imprisonment rose from 94 per 100 000 of the population in 1968 to 153 per 100 000 in 1981. This dramatic increase is all the more startling given that the prison population had been virtually constant in the preceding thirteen years. The US prison population in

January 1988 was 531 609 while the imprisonment rate was 228 per 100 000 (*New York Times*, 25 April, 1988).

In addition to statistical analyses of population trends there are an increasing number of studies designed to collect information about individuals' careers through the various institutions. Some have been based on institutional records while others have been based on interviews with individuals who have been diagnosed as mentally ill and were in jail at the time of the interview.

The process of de-institutionalization occurred across the US at more or less the same time. The factors which lead to hospital closures are described below. Analysis of the data shows that the process of closing the mental hospitals fell into two distinct phases. In the first phase, state mental hospitals were run down by discharging long-stay patients into the community and by giving early discharges to newly admitted patients. During this phase, the state mental hospitals provided back-up for the new community facilities. In the second phase, something entirely novel happened, changes in legislation and psychiatric practice coincided to produce a decline in hospital admissions and the tendency for hospitals to be used only for short periods to stabilize patients after crises. Steadman & Morrissey (1987) call these phases 'opening the back doors' and 'closing the front doors' respectively.

The precise reasons for these changes vary slightly according to the different sources. Gudeman & Shore (1984) suggest that de-institutionalization has been assisted by new forms of medication, concern for the civil rights of institutionalized persons, and the arrival of a political ideology which favoured fewer restrictions on individuals. Adler (1986) adds that, in many states, the criteria for admitting patients involuntarily had become more stringent while the criteria for discharge became less onerous. A significant shift in the funding arrangements for the mentally ill coincided with these legal and political changes, federal money was made available to match state funds for community care but not for running hospitals (Gudeman & Shore, 1984).

That briefly is the 'transcarceration' hypothesis, but what is the evidence for it? The hypothesis involves two separate populations. The first consists of those people who were in mental hospitals before the process of de-institutionalization began but who are now in prisons. The second consists of the group who are mentally ill and have never had any contact with the mental health system and who are imprisoned if they now commit offences. Most of the research to date has concentrated on the former group. The consensus emerging from research in the US is that, while prison populations have increased dramatically, there seems to have been no switching of populations directly to the prisons from the state mental hospitals. What seems more likely is that the impact of de-institutionalization on the criminal justice system is actually on the local jails, not on the state prisons. Jails hold prisoners pre-trial and sub-sequently, if they are convicted of a misdemeanour, for sentences of up to one year. The argument is that individuals released from mental hospitals live in run-down areas of large cities and, if they engage in disturbed behaviour, they are likely to be reported to the police and end up being sentenced for minor acts of nuisance.

Has a similar process been occurring in England and Wales? We have had a policy of community care since 1959, and we have seen both a decline in the mental hospital population and an increasing prison population. Some medical spokesmen have suggested that the same de-institutionalization process is happening here. In their evidence to the House of Commons Social Services Committee, inquiring into the Prison Medical Service, both Doctors Kilgour and Hindson stated that they knew of people who had formerly been in mental hospitals now appearing in the prisons (House of Commons, 1985: Q77A & Q188A). This could equally well be interpreted as the criminalization of the mentally ill (see below) as much as part of the 'transcarceration' hypothesis. More recently, Dr Weller and his co-author Diana Brahams restated Lionel Penrose's view that there is an inverse relationship between the number of psychiatric beds and the prison population, and they described how the process of transfer could occur as a result of inadequate community care (Brahams & Weller, 1985*a*). The concern was voiced more recently in the debate following the House of Commons statement on Community Care in July 1989. Nicholas Winterton MP asked the Secretary of State how he would ensure that mentally ill people did not end up in prison because of the inadequacy of community facilities (House of Commons Debates, 12 July 1989, col. 986).

But what of the evidence provided by changes in institutional popu-lations? The prison population in England and Wales has been rising continuously over the years and the mental hospital population has been declining, as seen in Fig. 5.1. The trends seen in the institutional populations in England and Wales are similar to those described in the American literature. The prison population rose from 31 063 in 1962 to 46 974 in 1986 while the mental hospital population fell from 134 763 to 64 921 in the same period. In 1986, the prison population was 51% greater than it had been in 1962 while the total number of mental hospital

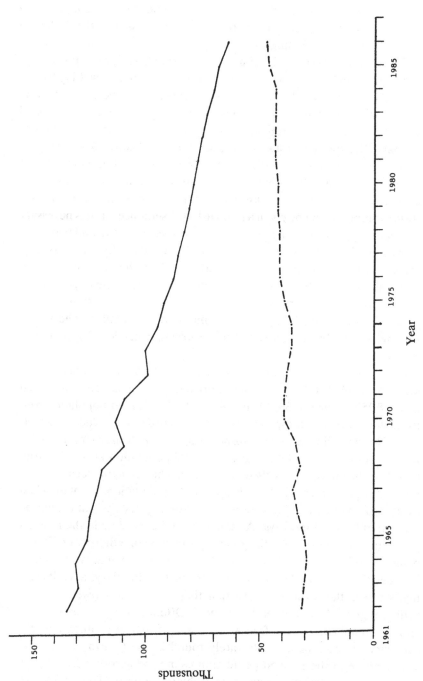

Fig. 5.1. Prison population and mental hospital residents in England and Wales 1962–1986. ———— Mental hospital residents.
-·-·- Prison population.

residents was 52% less than in 1962. The number of people involved in the increase in the prison population is however less than the decline in the mental hospital population.

But gross trends conceal as much as they reveal. The prison population is composed of two distinct sub-groups, those on remand awaiting trial or sentence and those who have been sentenced, and these ought to be looked at separately. The rationale for doing so is that mentally ill offenders might well be remanded in custody to ensure their appearance at trial in the absence of stable accommodation outside or for psychiatric reports to be prepared if the individual's behaviour is perceived as unusual. The mentally ill may appear disproportionately in the remand population when charged with comparatively minor offences but as a result of reports may be given a non-custodial sentence.[2] If it is necessary to disaggregate the prison population it is also necessary to add two other groups to the other side of the equation. Community care has also involved the mental handicap hospitals; people with a mental handicap might also contribute to the offender population after discharge into the community. The picture is further complicated by the existence of the special hospitals which might absorb mentally ill offenders who would otherwise have been imprisoned if the 'transcarceration' hypothesis is correct.

Information on the relative movements of these five groups is presented in Table 5.1.[3] The number of prisoners under sentence increased from 28 258 in 1962 to 36 655 in 1986 while the remand population rose from 2805 to 10 319 in the same period; rises of 30% and 268% respectively. Not only did the mental hospital population decline (from 134 763 to 64 921) but the mental handicap hospital population also fell – from 61 471 in 1962 to 35 942 in 1986, a 41% fall. The dramatic decline in the mental hospital and mental handicap hospital populations is not matched by an equally dramatic increase in the prison population that cannot be accounted for in other ways. A large part in the increase in the remand population has been due to the greater proportion of either-way offences being committed to the Crown Court for trial. This category of offence includes the moderately serious offences such as burglary, assaults and thefts where the justices believe that their sentencing powers are not sufficient given the nature of the offences. Offences such as minor acts of criminal damage, benefit frauds, and shoplifting, are either entirely summary offences or are only rarely found in the Crown Court lists. The increase in the remand population cannot be accounted for by an increase in prisoners remanded for psychiatric reports. The number of

Table 5.1. *Prison population and mental hospital residents, 1962–86*

Population/residents	1962	1966 Change	1971 Change	1976 Change	1981 Change	1986 Change
Prisoners under sentence	28 258 (100)	29 527 (104)	34 576 (122)	35 838 (127)	36 022 (127)	36 655 (130)
Prisoners on remand	2805 (100)	3559 (127)	5133 (183)	5602 (200)	7289 (260)	10 319 (368)
Mental hospital patients	134 763 (100)	124 160 (92)	109 749 (81)	88 947 (66)	77 574 (58)	64 921 (48)
Special hospital patients	2148 (100)	2142 (100)	2242 (104)	2181 (102)	1791 (83)	1694 (79)
Mental handicap patients	61 471 (100)	64 694 (105)	54 409 (89)	51 100 (83)	45 253 (74)	35 992 (59)

Note: The figure in brackets represents the percentage change in the annual figure compared with the 1962 baseline.

Table 5.2. *Receptions to prison and admissions to mental hospitals, 1962–86*

Receptions/admissions	1962	1966 Change	1971 Change	1976 Change	1981 Change	1986 Change
Prisoners under sentence	53 603 (100)	62 787 (117)	60 429 (113)	68 479 (128)	88 110 (164)	86 153 (161)
Prisoners on remand	58 994 (100)	67 668 (115)	82 064 (139)	78 836 (134)	74 818 (127)	75 657 (128)
Mental hospital patients	148 671 (100)	166 272 (112)	173 230 (117)	190 262 (129)	197 592 (133)	210 665 (142)
Special hospital patients	NA*	203 (100)	384 (189)	236 (116)	282 (107)	234 (115)
Mental handicap hospital patients	8087 (100)	9511 (118)	11 193 (138)	15 122 (187)	23 758 (294)	39 739 (491)

* Admission figures for the Special Hospitals were not included in the *Annual Report for 1962* of the Ministry of Health.

remands for psychiatric reports has changed significantly over the years. In 1960, about 6000 reports were prepared. The demand for reports peaked at nearly 14 000 in 1970, and has fallen away progressively ever since (Watson, 1986). In the years 1983 to 1985 the numbers of reports were 8923, 9893 and 7689 respectively. A further point to be made about these institutional population figures is that they relate only to part of the de-institutionalization process termed 'opening the back doors'; what is also needed is knowledge about admissions.

Table 5.2 provides information on receptions and admissions since 1962.[4] There have been large increases in receptions into prisons for prisoners under sentence and on remand. Receptions of prisoners under sentence rose from 53 603 in 1962 to 86 153 in 1986; an increase of 61%. The comparable figures for remand receptions are 58 994 and 75 657 respectively; a 28% increase. Admissions to mental hospitals and mental handicap hospitals have also risen. The rise in admissions to mental handicap hospitals is particularly dramatic – from 8087 to 39 739 over the same time period, an increase of 391%. Admissions to mental hospitals also rose, but not so spectacularly, from 148 671 to 210 665, or 42%. If the population and reception figures for prison are increasing, then the average length of stay in prison is getting longer. On the other hand, a falling number of residents in mental hospitals and mental handicap hospitals together with a rising number of admissions means that the average stay is getting shorter. These conclusions are consistent with what we know from other sources such as judicial statistics and statements of policy on the use of mental handicap hospitals for respite care and the use of psychiatric facilities for short-term crisis intervention work. This information provides a significant contrast with what happened in the US where admissions to mental hospitals declined as rapidly as the mental hospital population. Mental hospitals in Britain are still accepting patients. It is not yet clear whether we have yet to reach the 'closing the front door' phase, as the main programme of mental hospital closures is a year or two away. The other point to be made is that the reduction in length of stay in the mental hospitals probably means that psychiatrists are becoming increasingly selective in their admission practices. Anyone needing longer-term care may simply not be admitted to the acute units based in district hospitals which are not orientated towards that type of care.

The American analyses of the 'transcarceration' hypothesis are fairly sophisticated methodologically, for example, Steadman and his colleagues carried out comparisons of trends in states with different patterns of change, but nowhere do they mention the sex ratios of institutional populations (Steadman *et al.*, 1984). One of the basic assumptions underlying British discussions of institutional populations is that women make up a small proportion of the prison population but they make up a much larger proportion, the majority, of the mental hospital population. If the 'transcarceration' hypothesis is correct then the relative increase of the female prison population should be greater than that for men as the number of women who can be released from the mental hospitals is so much greater.

Table 5.3 provides similar information to that in Table 5.1 but divides each institutional population by sex.[5] In addition to the actual figures there is also an indication of the extent of change relative to 1962. If one considers the mental hospital and mental handicap hospital figures first it is noticeable that the trend is virtually the same for both men and women. The policies pursued in mental hospitals have meant that in 1986 the sex ratio was almost the same as it had been in 1962: 42% male and 58% female. The sex ratio in mental handicap hospitals also remained constant at about 55% male and 45% female. Women comprise a very small part of both the sentenced and remand populations of prisons, about 5%. This proportion remained the same in 1986 even though there was a greater proportionate increase in female prisoners under sentence than males. Although the number of women prisoners on remand has more than doubled, that change is dwarfed by the trebling of the male remand population.

It should also be noted that these changes in the prisons did not occur at such a constant rate as that found in the mental hospitals and the mental handicap hospitals. The population of sentenced male prisoners has been virtually constant since 1971, and there was an 18% increase in the period 1966–1971. The number of women prisoners under sentence fell between 1962 and 1971 and there have been two increases of over 25% since then (i.e. 1971–76 and 1981–86). Among remand prisoners the pace of change has been greater but the increase has been more marked among the male prisoners. There does not seem to have been a massive switch of women from mental hospitals to the prisons.

It is essential to look at male and female reception/admission figures in light of the earlier general discussion of receptions and admissions. Table 5.4 provides information on the sex of receptions/admissions. The 1986

Table 5.3. *Prison population and mental hospital residents by sex, 1962–86*

Population/residents		1962	1966 Change	1971 Change	1976 Change	1981 Change	1986 Change
Prisoners under sentence	Male	27 433 (100)	28 764 (105)	33 780 (123)	34 852 (127)	34 940 (127)	35 358 (129)
	Female	825 (100)	763 (92)	796 (96)	986 (120)	1082 (131)	1297 (157)
Prisoners on remand	Male	2633 (100)	3363 (128)	4893 (185)	5306 (202)	6964 (264)	9883 (375)
	Female	172 (100)	196 (114)	240 (140)	296 (172)	325 (189)	436 (253)
Mental hospitals	Male	57 800 (100)	53 787 (93)	47 654 (82)	35 946 (62)	30 600 (53)	25 500 (44)
	Female	76 963 (100)	70 373 (91)	62 095 (81)	47 993 (62)	42 600 (55)	34 800 (45)
Special hospitals	Male	1601 (100)	1641 (102)	1749 (109)	NA —	NA —	NA —
	Female	547 (100)	501 (92)	493 (90)	NA —	NA —	NA —
Mental handicap hospitals	Male	33 433 (100)	34 935 (104)	29 734 (89)	26 946 (81)	23 900 (71)	19 000 (57)
	Female	28 038 (100)	29 759 (106)	24 675 (88)	21 827 (78)	19 200 (68)	15 200 (54)

Table 5.4. *Receptions to prison and admissions to mental hospitals by sex, 1962–86*

Receptions/admissions		1962	1966 Change	1971 Change	1976 Change	1981 Change	1986 Change
Prisoners under sentence	Male	50 767 (100)	60 169 (119)	58 423 (115)	65 800 (130)	84 196 (166)	81 933 (161)
	Female	2836 (100)	2618 (83)	2006 (71)	2679 (94)	3914 (138)	4220 (149)
Prisoners on remand	Male	54 721 (100)	63 680 (116)	77 550 (142)	74 061 (135)	70 547 (129)	71 880 (131)
	Female	4273 (100)	3988 (93)	4514 (106)	4775 (112)	4271 (100)	3777 (88)
Mental hospitals	Male	59 982 (100)	67 985 (113)	70 763 (118)	77 078 (129)	79 826 (133)	89 473 (149)
	Female	88 689 (100)	98 287 (111)	102 467 (116)	113 184 (128)	117 766 (133)	121 192 (137)
Special hospitals	Male	NA —	187 (100)	302 (161)	190 (102)	250 (134)	NA —
	Female	NA —	16 (100)	82 (513)	46 (288)	32 (200)	NA —
Mental handicap hospitals	Male	4529 (100)	5320 (117)	6122 (135)	8517 (189)	13 144 (290)	21 674 (479)
	Female	3558 (100)	4191 (118)	5071 (143)	6605 (186)	10 614 (298)	18 065 (508)

figures show increases in all categories bar one (women remand prisoners). Receptions of both male and female prisoners increased but the increase in receptions of male prisoners was greater than for women. The increase for male prisoners has been fairly steady but for women the increase is of comparatively recent origin, it began in the 1976–81 period. The picture for remand prisoners is more confused. The number of remands of male prisoners peaked in 1971 and seems to have reached a plateau at a level 30% higher than in 1962. The trend among women remand prisoners is significant as it shows the only fall at the end of the period under study. This fall follows a series of fluctuations, but the fall since 1976 is 25%.

When attention is turned to the mental hospitals, the increases in receptions of male and female patients are almost always in step. The only divergence from this pattern is in the final period when the rate of admissions of male patients was greater than that for women. The largest changes of all are to be found in admissions to mental handicap hospitals where the rate of increase has risen significantly since 1981.

There seems to be little unequivocal evidence from these data to support the 'transcarceration' hypothesis in England and Wales since 1962. The most that can be said on this evidence is that on the one hand there have been significant increases in the populations of female prisoners (both on remand and under sentence) and in the population of male prisoners on remand, while on the other hand, the populations of mental illness and mental handicap hospitals have fallen dramatically. There is little hard evidence to suggest a cross-over of people from mental hospitals to prisons.

There are a number of good reasons for not being able to sustain the 'transcarceration' hypothesis.

(a) The mental hospitals have been run down but the full-blooded closure programme is still in its relatively early stages and its effects will not be felt for some time to come. Those remaining in the mental hospitals are unlikely to be of the age and sex normally associated with crime, but it is not possible to obtain comparable age distributions for prison populations and hospital residents.

(b) The former patients who are discharged from long-stay mental hospitals may be defined officially as living in the community but that may only mean that they are in the wards of a privately owned nursing home. The 'community' is any hospital/home not owned by the NHS.

(c) Official statistical publications are of little help with this sort of analysis. Some support for the 'transcarceration' hypothesis might be given if more former mental hospital patients were being received into prison leading to changes in the age structure of the prisons, but the prison statistics are only concerned with age in so far as it reflects the legal differences between youth custody and adult imprisonment.

(d) The sentenced prison population is serving longer rather than shorter sentences. There does not seem to have been an influx of people convicted of the minor nuisance type offences.

The criminalization of the mentally ill

What sorts of mechanisms might lead to the criminalization of the mentally ill? At least three possibilities can be specified:

(a) There may simply be more mentally ill people in the community who are at risk of committing offences. This class of people might include two separate groups – those who have previously been in mental hospitals but who have been discharged into the community and those people who, although mentally ill, have never been in contact with the psychiatric services.

(b) The police may be reluctant to process mentally ill offenders through the mental health services for either of the following reasons:
  (i) previous difficulties with health and social services staff;
  (ii) inability/unwillingness to recognize that offenders may be mentally ill.

(c) The courts may not recognize or accept that an offender is mentally ill. The court may not ask for reports to be prepared on the offender or may not accept their conclusions. The prison medical officer responsible for preparing the report may decide that the offender is not mentally ill, or alternatively he may diagnose mental illness, but may not be able to persuade a mental hospital to accept the offender on a hospital order. Some offenders remanded on bail have in the past been refused contact with psychiatrists who would not accept individuals whom they could not treat until the offender had been sentenced.

All three of these possible routes may lead to more mentally ill people ending up in prisons or at least they may be taken as hypothetical routes to prison. What evidence is there to accept or reject them?

If we start with the police, who are the initial gate-keepers to the criminal justice system, the evidence is mixed. Sims and Symonds (1975) reported that they had evidence that in the previous decade the police in and around Birmingham had increased referrals to the mental health service. They argued that, in the period under study (1962–73), the police seemed to have become more rather than less willing to be involved with the mentally ill and to view incidents as the result of mental illness.

It is not clear whether the same could be said now. Under the terms of *Police and Criminal Evidence Act* 1984 and its Codes of Practice, there are special provisions to protect categories of suspects, including the mentally ill or handicapped. The *Police and Criminal Evidence Act* defines mental handicap but not mental illness. The Codes of Practice leave it to the judgement of the custody officer whether the suspect is, or may be, mentally ill. An 'appropriate adult' would then be asked to attend the station while the mentally ill individual is questioned. The protections built into the 1984 Act are stronger than those found in the previous Judges' Rules. In recently published research, David Brown has argued that:

The net effect of the custody officer's duties in relation to juveniles and the mentally ill or handicapped may be to entail more work, case for case than for other prisoners, both in terms of more intensive supervision and in contacting appropriate persons. Special care may be needed in proceeding with investigation, particuarly interrogation, with these detainees.

(Brown, 1989: p. 38)

In the police stations under study, Brown found that 1% of those detained were recorded as mentally ill or handicapped. The types of offences for which the mentally ill and handicapped were detained were different from those for which other suspects were held. The mentally ill and handicapped were less frequently arrested for crime; the largest single group (43%) had been reported as missing persons by relatives or institutions. Nearly a quarter (22%) were arrested as a result of offences of criminal damage (Brown, 1989, *ibid*).

In a recent review of police/social work interactions, Stephen (1988) has argued that the police frequently complain that they are often unable to get a social worker to attend a police station quickly, especially if the request should be made outside normal office hours. Stephen quotes a comment by the Police Superintendents' Association to the effect that duty social workers are loath to respond to emergency calls outside their own area of competence, and if they do attend they are then thought to behave less than competently.

The use of police cells to hold remand prisoners has also been the subject of criticism by serving police officers. Boothroyd (1988) quotes a Parliamentary Written Answer by Mr John Patten, Home Office Minister, stating that on the night of 6/7 December 1987, 51 remand prisoners were being held in police cells while awaiting psychiatric reports. No one would suggest that police cells were at all adequate for anything but the shortest period of detention; the police are not trained or equipped to cope with mentally ill prisoners. The reality has been that police cells were used for longer-term remands. Boothroyd cites cases of individuals spending up to three months on the road before finally being admitted to some more settled accommodation.

If mentally ill people are admitted to a remand prison what are their chances of being accepted by a hospital on an in-patient or out-patient basis for treatment? On this point, the evidence seems mixed. When Taylor and Gunn (1984a) undertook their fieldwork in 1979/80 police cells were not being used to accommodate remand prisoners. They argued that the prevalence of symptoms of psychotic disorders on entry into prison was high, 9% of the sample. Taylor and Gunn reported that a large proportion (45%) of those diagnosed as schizophrenic had been charged with a violent offence. The authors then go on to say

This tends to imply that the population of this remand prison was unnecessarily inflated by the bringing of criminal charges against men who showed minor disturbances in behaviour but were ill and perhaps should have been in hospital.

(*ibid*: p. 1948)

At the same time the authors suggest that 'A balancing effect is that many sick offenders are still dealt with without recourse to courts' (*ibid*).

When it comes to the question of how remand prisoners were dealt with, Taylor and Gunn reported that those charged with offences of personal violence were least likely to be convicted. The authors suggested that the police tend to view mentally ill men as more dangerous than the people they regard as psychiatrically normal. Taylor and Gunn then say that other factors may lead to mentally ill offenders being remanded in custody, e.g. homelessness; consequently there is no evidence that the mentally ill were particularly vulnerable to involvement in the criminal justice system.

Taylor and Gunn also argue that their study did not support the idea that psychiatric remands did little to help the mentally ill. About a third of the mentally ill offenders who were convicted were given hospital orders. The most important factor militating against acceptance into a hospital is the presence of complicating problems such as substance abuse or some additional diagnosis. The belief that violence leads to rejection was not supported and 'if anything, a history of violence improved their chances of receiving a hospital order.' (Taylor & Gunn, 1984b: p.12)

More recently Coid (1988a,b) has published the results of a retro-spective study of all mentally abnormal men remanded to Winchester prison for psychiatric reports in the years 1979–83. Coid focused on both the process by which a decision to offer treatment was made and the extent to which NHS psychiatrists were prepared to offer treatment. Eighty-hree out of 388 men in the sample were refused treatment. Coid states:

These generally were the men most in need of care and exhibiting the severest degree of social impairment, which is the cause for great concern. Furthermore, the findings support those of another study (Robertson, 1982) suggesting that these men are a sub-group of mentally handicapped subjects no longer admitted to NHS hospitals when they exhibit deviant behaviour.

(Coid, 1988a: p. 1781)

Coid states that the rejected men posed the least threat to the community in terms of their criminal behaviour.

Significantly Coid then looks at the characteristics of decision-makers which he believes are related to the various outcomes. Consultants from older style mental hospitals were more likely to accept prisoners, particu-larly on hospital orders, than were consultants from district general hospitals and prestigious academic units, 'especially those espousing a community based, rather than hospital based approach' (Coid, 1988a: p. 1782). One part of the admission problem may have been consensus style management in the hospital where a dissenting vote by one member of the team is effectively a veto.

Coid concludes that many of the men fell through the gap between open wards and community programmes, on the one hand, and the regional secure units and special hospitals on the other. These individuals find it difficult to survive in the community, and often being homeless they quickly come to the attention of the police:

By finding their way into prison many are obtaining the only care and treatment that anyone is prepared to offer them.

(Coid 1988a: p. 1782)

These two studies are important for several reasons. First, they are rare examples of empirical investigation of this vexed issue. Second, Coid's work helps to illuminate the process that Taylor and Gunn were describing. But both suffer from unfortunate deficiencies. The Taylor and Gunn article contains no reference to the previous institutional careers of the sample. This is an unfortunate omission, given the authors' references to the problem of what was happening to the mentally ill caught up in the criminal justice system. The information contained in records was incomplete and too unreliable to be used in their analysis. Some reliable data on previous involvement with the mental health services would have prevented the sort of inference drawn by Brahams and Weller from the Taylor and Gunn study, namely that finding an over-representation of schizophrenics of 22½ times population based expectations was the result of fewer psychiatric hospital places and hospital discharge policies (Brahams & Weller, 1985b). We simply do not know where these men had been before. Nor do we know whether the situation was better or worse in 1979–80 than in previous or subsequent years.

Coid's study is an interesting addition to the literature as he concentrates on the selection process as well as its outcomes. Significantly Coid draws our attention to the differences between regional health authorities and their policies and operational practices. The Oxford Regional Health Authority did not (at that time) have either a secure unit or a forensic psychiatrist, unlike Wessex Regional Health Authority which provided the comparison. These organizational differences have implications for any macro-level analysis of population shifts: historically the regional health authorities have changed at different times and in different ways and consequently the impacts of community care policies will have been neither uniform nor synchronous.

A comparison of the studies by Coid and Taylor and Gunn throws up the interesting question of rejection rates. Coid clearly feels that the 30% rejection rate in the Oxford Regional Health Authority is too high both absolutely and by comparison with the 16% rejection rate in Wessex. Less than a third of the Taylor and Gunn sample received a hospital order. It would have been useful to have had a Coid style organizational analysis for Taylor and Gunn's sample. Not all of those rejected by the mental health services were sentenced to imprisonment; other outcomes are possible but it is not clear what distinguishes those who are imprisoned.

Conclusions

Even after this analysis has been presented it is difficult to draw any hard conclusions. There has been a significant change in institutional populations over the past 20 years: prison populations have risen while mental hospital populations have declined. But there is no real evidence to suggest that large numbers of former mental hospital patients are now in the prisons. The process of community care moved the most able mental hospital patients into the community first. The older, the more frail, and possibly more institutionalized have been left until later and they have frequently been moved into other forms of residential care. The young men who form the greater part of the prison population were not to be found in mental hospitals in large numbers to begin with, although it is possible to speculate that they may have made up a significant proportion of the mental handicap hospital population. This is not to deny that there may be mentally ill young men coming into prison who have never been in contact with the mental health services or who may have been rejected by those services for being too disruptive or too violent.

The second hypothesis examined raised the possibility that mentally ill people may now be more likely than before to be criminalized. The research on the effects of the *Police and Criminal Evidence Act* is disturbing suggesting as it does that the police may, for the first time, have good reasons for not considering a suspect to be mentally ill. Just how widespread this problem is remains to be seen.

Notes

1. I would like to thank my colleagues John Brown, Maggie Clifton and Ian Shaw for their helpful comments on an earlier version of this paper.
2. The table in the Annual Reports of the Prison Department which include the number of medical and psychiatric reports is no longer presented in the new style Annual Reports.
3. The data presented in these tables are drawn from the Annual Reports of the Prison Department and Annual Reports of the Ministry of Health. After 1968, the figures for mental hospitals became more difficult to find and in the mid 1970s the annual Health and Personal Social Service Statistics are published separately for England and Wales. Consistency over time has suffered considerably as can be seen from the tables.
4. Admission figures for the special hospitals were not included in the Annual Report for 1962 of the Ministry of Health.
5. The published data on residents of special hospitals do not include information on sex of residents.

6

New directions for service provision: a personal view

P. BOWDEN

In 1939 Lionel Penrose published an incidental finding in an investigation whose primary purpose was to ascertain the meanings of the terms 'insanity' and 'mental deficiency' in different parts of the world (Penrose, 1939). His views were based on two assumptions: the first was the 'knowledge' based on Cyril Burt's *The Young Delinquent* that mental disorder predisposed to crime; the second was the 'supposition' that the criminal population contained a group who should properly be labelled as mentally diseased (Burt, 1925).

Penrose said that generally there were two ways of segregating the socially undesirable: wait until a crime is committed and then remove them from society; provide institutional care as material for 'medical attention'. He emphasized the view that medical attention would be judged by its success in preventing damage to the community from crime.

Penrose considered the larger European countries in the year 1934. (For the present discussion three countries have been chosen because of their similar populations in 1934 of about 40 million.) He did not question the reliability and validity of his criterion groups: mental disease was measured by the number of institutional beds in a country; crime by the amount of prison accommodation.

Although the claim was unfounded Penrose concluded:

. . . there is a definite incompatibility between the development of mental health services and the need for accommodation in prisons.

Penrose then returned to his social hygiene theory. He suggested that attention to mental health may help to prevent the occurrence of serious

78

Table 6.1. *Mentally diseased inmates and prison populations in 1934 (Penrose, 1939)*

Country	Number of mentally diseased inmates/ 1000 population	Number of prisoners/ 1000 population
England and Wales	4.72	0.3
France	2.31	0.56
Italy	1.97	1.26

Table 6.2. *Mentally diseased inmates and crime rates in 1934 (Penrose, 1939)*

Country	Number of mentally diseased inmates/1000 population	Number of convictions for serious offences/ 1000 population	Murder/million population
England and Wales	4.76	1.6	6
France	2.31	4.3	10
Italy	1.97	3.4	23

crimes, particularly deliberate homicide. He drew the inference from the figures set out in Table 6.2.

Whatever caution Penrose showed in interpreting his findings in 1939 had disappeared by 1943 when he wrote in the *American Journal of Mental Deficiency* on the statistical relationship between mental deficiency and crime:

... the European statistics suggest strongly that attention to the problems of mental health actually assists in preventing crime.

(Penrose, 1943)

And:

The prevalence of serious crimes, especially those which imply violence against the person, appears to be much more marked in countries which provide relatively few beds for mental patients.

Penrose stated unequivocally that attention to mental hygiene made an 'important' contribution to the prevention of crime in the community.

Of course the amount of crime and mental disease in a community cannot be measured by looking at the numbers in mental institutions and prisons. And drawing an inference about the criterion groups from a seeming inverse relationship between them is unwarranted. The same criticisms hold for Penrose's assumptions made from the 'serious crime offences' and 'murder' figures: despite his assertion to the contrary he failed to show that attention to mental hygiene made any contribution to the prevention of crime.

The superficial attractiveness of Penrose's speculations led to the designation 'law' despite his inability to show a constant order between the criterion groups. Neither did he provide a scientific explanation of the relationship he believed to exist, even less one which carried with it an inevitability or a high degree of probability that it would hold good in future or hypothetical situations.

The most recent adherents of the Penrose School are the Wellers. Writing in *Medicine, Science and the Law* in 1988 they tease:

Since 1954, 75 000 patients have been discharged from long-stay beds in psychiatric hospitals. Where have they all gone? – those that are not dead that is.
(Weller & Weller, 1988).

Not to local authorities' diminishing resources. Hospital or prison they ask? It is clear from the onset that the Wellers know the answer and they turn to the Director of the Prison Medical Service to support their view:

. . . The proportion of prisoners harbouring psychopathology is rising as well as the severity of that pathology.
(Kilgour, 1984)

(It is as if psychopathology was a disease.)

By selective juxtaposition the Wellers suggest an association. First the increase in the prison population is highlighted and then?

Meanwhile the number of patients who occupy long-stay beds in psychiatric hospitals continues to fall . . .
(*ibid*)

The Wellers plotted residents in psychiatric hospitals 1950–1984 against the number of prison inmates. They found a straight line best fit, and a correlation coefficient of 0.94. They comment:

Of course, an association does not establish a causal relationship but it is difficult to put forward convincing explanations for this exceedingly strong relationship, probably unprecedented in demographic data, except by postulating that there is some decanting from the psychiatric hospitals to the prisons.

(*ibid*)

'Some decanting' appears a cautious comment but in his 1989 *Nature* article Weller Senior piles assumption on assumption:

This cannot be an auspicious time simultaneously to close 55 psychiatric hospitals in England ... can it be mere coincidence that the British Government is also planning to open 26 new prisons, one on the site of the recently closed Banstead Psychiatric Hospital.

(Weller, 1989)

The irony is powerful and the Penrose Law has achieved the status of popular mythology.

Maxwell's guide to elementary statistics provides some enlightenment. Maxwell pointed out that a correlation coefficient is a measure of concomitant agreement between pairs of scores on two variables:

... the coefficient itself is just an index of agreement and on its own supplies no information about the reasons why the variables are related ... The late Professor Udny Yule, for instance, reported a significant correlation between the number of apples imported into Great Britain and the numbers of divorces in each of a series of years.'

(Maxwell, 1970)

Following Walker's critical summary *Behaviour and Misbehaviour: Explanations and Non-Explanations* what Penrose supplied was an analogy (Walker, 1977). Penrose suggested that the phenomena he studied obeyed a generalization as if a particular mechanism was in operation. What is that generalization? The suggestion appears to have been that there was a relatively stable mass of individuals who were in one form of environment, asylums, rather than another, prison. The two were used interchangeably. The benefit of the asylum was its effect on reducing crime.

The Wellers support Penrose's argument and carry it further. The community is replete with individuals who were once in hospitals. De-institutionalization is not the only villain: lack of a community treatment order and the flight into fine (neurosis and talking treatments) as opposed to coarse (psychosis) psychiatry are also responsible.

What is the general mechanism linking asylum and prison? It seems that what is proposed is that behaviour reflecting mental disorder can either be criminalized or medicalized. If it is not medicalized it is criminalized although the reverse is not the case. It follows that, if long-term (?) institutions were provided for 100 000 or so souls, there would be quantitatively and qualitatively less 'psychopathology' in prison. This writer's view is that the analogy remains unproven as is the existence of an interchangeable mechanism between asylum and prison.

This scepticism is based on lack of evidence in several areas: showing that there are significant numbers of prisoners who would have been in hospital before but are not now; showing that there has been a shift of individuals from hospital to prison; showing that there are significant numbers of prisoners who should be in hospital but are not.

What follows is a direct quotation from a book which provides an answer. The author discusses the failure of the community to care for their mentally ill brethren:

So with almost reckless enthusiasm the gates of the mental hospitals were flung open and a horde of mental cripples, unable to survive in society without considerable support, were discharged only to find that this support either did not exist or was hopelessly inadequate. Some in order to meet the primitive urge to survive stole food from shops . . . the ping-pong sequence now begins, or in many cases is continued . . . they are fed back under the provisions of the 1959 Act from the prison system into the mental hospital system only to be discharged, or allowed to discharge themselves, or to abscond. The whole sequence is repeated and the 'open door', a concomitant of the progressive hospital, is thus in effect transmuted into the 'revolving door'.

(Rollin, 1969)

The quotation is, of course, from Rollin's book *The Mentally Abnormal Offender and the Law*. What Rollin said is very significant: it was not the decline of the mental hospital which led to the translocation of large numbers of chronic psychotics into the community, it was their opening in the first place. Rollin discusses the process at Horton Hospital:

In 1938 the 'escapes' of male patients from Horton . . . recorded in meticulous detail . . . numbered exactly eight, . . . security in those days was one of the hallmarks of an efficient mental hospital and, judged by this criterion, Horton must have been highly regarded.

(*ibid*)

Rollin then describes events after the war.

... with a great sense of urgency, ward doors were unlocked and blocks removed from windows ... the hideous railings which fenced in the airing courts ... were at last torn down ... as freedom came in through the open doors, security went out through the windows.

(ibid)

From the figure of eight abscondences in 1938 Rollin gave the numbers for 1961 and 1962. In 1961, of 207 offenders admitted, 48% absconded, in 1962, 52%. Taking both years there was a total of 235 abcondences. Rollin considered that half the absconders were either 'incurable or incorrigible', unsuitable for admission to any conventional mental hospital **without bars** (my emphasis).

These considerations lead to the conclusion that is was the opening up of large mental hospitals which led to the translocation of chronic psychotics into the community. That they have been relocated in prison remains unproven. To relocate them in medical facilities would require large scale detention.

Many of the difficulties which bedevil discussion in this area are caused by simplistic views or polarizations. Furthermore data is interpreted in ways which are completely beyond the scope of the original enquiry. Diagnosis is seen as a fixed and unitary concept; a label makes 'a case' and through some moral imperative the conclusion is drawn that the labelled should be in treatment, in hospital, or subject to community care. Reputations can be made by assuming a high moral stand in these matters. No account is taken of a person's personality or of habits such as drug and alcohol abuse. To say that a person is, or was, schizophrenic means little when the added factors of, say, a sociopathic personality and a dependence on alcohol are omitted. The person's attitude to treatment is also important. Non-compliant psychotics can only be treated in the short-term. The individual's own wishes concerning where they want to live also have to be taken into account. Rollin's patients voted with their feet: they did not want what was on offer and absconded, however irrational that choice might seem. Freedom includes the ability to choose what is undesirable and damaging as well as what is advantageous and wholesome. The last point is that each case must be decided on the prevailing circumstances. A single disposal, appropriate at all points in a person's psychiatric and criminal career cannot be prescribed.

The present author's view is that there are very few people in prison who could be engaged in treatment elsewhere without a wholesale return to a closed asylum system. In fact, the numbers are so few that it is impossible to draw any general conclusions from them regarding their needs in terms of general service provision. Where there are mentally ill people in prison, they are characterized overwhelmingly by anti-social personalities, substance abuse, non-compliance, and the simple wish not to be 'in treatment'.

If this vignette is accurate, we are forced to recognize the necessity of improving the treatment of the mentally ill in prisons. Using the 'flood-gates' metaphor the Home Office appears to be motivated by the belief that once responsibility for the mentally ill in prisons is accepted – rather than saying it lies with the NHS – prisons will be inundated by courts sentencing chronic psychotics to receive treatment in custody. This over-used and inaccurate characterization of NHS psychiatry as reneging on its responsibility to provide treatment for mentally ill offenders is an excuse for doing nothing.

Prisons must accept that the chronic mentally ill will always be with them. A statutory basis for the treatment of mentally ill in prisons is required urgently; the present consent to treatment practices are unwork-able and regressive. Conditions too must be changed and it is hardly believable that prison doctors continue to allow psychotic patients to be contained in 'special medical rooms'. A consultant psychiatrist working at Brixton Prison in 1989 wrote:

These rooms are bare apart from a mattress, extremely dirty and often faeces-smeared as a result of the patient's mental state, and stiflingly hot in summer and cold in winter. Patients are often naked because of their mental condition and have only a canvas blanket with which to keep warm. They may remain in this condition for some considerable time.

(Herridge, 1989)

In his pre-Butler response to the revised Glancy Committee report in 1974, Peter Scott wrote of the importance of stimulating therapeutic endeavours within the prison system. Scott was uncharacteristically blunt:

It would perhaps help if approved parts of the prison system could be designated as hospitals . . . so hospital orders could be effected either in prison or hospital . . . The Prison Medical Service should merge with the National Health Service, and the forensic psychiatrists, instead of running esoteric little units in the health service, should treat patients in prison thus bringing a benevolent medical influence within the reach of any prisoner needing it . . .

(Scott, 1974)

Scott concluded:

... will (Lord Butler's Committee on Mentally Abnormal Offenders) look beyond immediate administrative difficulties and give us a bold lead which will enable the Home Office and DHSS to work together in developing the resources of the prison system?

(ibid)

We now know that it failed to do so.

Discussion

The discussion of the 'Transcarceration Hypothesis' initiated by Dr Fowles' and Dr Bowden's papers was marked by attempts to conceptualize and broadly quantify changes in the situations of mentally disordered offenders consequent upon the run down of the old large asylums and the development of the community care approach. In general, this discussion did not consist of polemics for and against the current policies, although great concern was shown for the contemporary plight of many mentally disordered offenders. Rather, it concerned the need to develop an accurate picture of what was happening on the ground, in order to facilitate more effective NHS, Home Office and social services planning.

The transcarceration hypothesis

Dr Fowles opened his comments by acknowledging that, unlike Dr Bowden, he had initially uncritically accepted the broad truth of the Penrose Hypothesis, a position which he now felt to be in doubt. He went on to reiterate the basic position he had presented in his paper; that statistical evidence did not support the existence of a gross transcarceration process. However, he wished this to be reconciled with the mass of anecdotal evidence which seemed to suggest many individual instances of such transcarceration. The key questions were whether the prison population had qualitatively changed in an accumulative way, particularly to contain more individuals with a history of contact with psychiatric services, and whether the mentally ill, especially the violent mentally ill, were being increasingly criminalized.

It was suggested that the rejection of a broad transcarceration hypothesis might be premature. The Wellers may have jumped the gun in claiming that such a situation obtained in the UK before this could be proved, but they might be right (Weller & Weller, 1988; Weller, 1989). There were more mentally ill amongst the homeless, it was claimed. Probation officers believe that many in prison are mentally vulnerable, if not 'sectionable', while the police claim that they are dealing with an increasing number of individuals with mental health problems. Finally, mental health organizations report an increasing tendency for the mentally ill to end up in prison. It might be hard to say whether the Wellers are right, but equally Dr Bowden may not be correct in his assertions. The Wellers' claim was not a myth but an unproven hypothesis.

Regarding the homeless, it was pointed out that it was a mistake to regard all individuals in this situation as necessarily mentally ill or criminal. Only a very small proportion of the homeless were convicted and sentenced by the courts. They were the victims of social policies that left them on the streets, and it would be useful to compare the situation in the UK with other countries with better social provision. It was reported that although a large proportion (about three-quarters) of the homeless seen by psychiatric services had histories of psychiatric hospitalization, fewer than 50% had criminal histories, and only a small proportion of these were being hospitalized at any one time. It was therefore inappropriate to infer from existence of these individuals that it was right to campaign for the retention of the large asylums, rather than for the provision of more adequate community care. Furthermore, a substantial contribution to the decline in psychiatric hospital populations has been mortality amongst older chronic patients.

With respect to the situation in the prisons, although it might be true that a large proportion of inmates had mental health problems, this did not mean that all these should be placed in a hospital setting. Further, there was a higher proportion of such individuals in the remand than in the sentenced population. It was also pointed out that Steadman's research in the US indicated that the absolute number of mentally ill had grown in an expanding prison population, such that the proportion remained more or less the same.

It was suggested that, although Dr Fowles had broken down the global figures for hospital and prison populations into constituent parts, such as the proportion of women in the populations, this had only been undertaken to see if a global transcarceration hypothesis could be sustained. However, there remained a question of whether there might be a smaller transcarcerated population, perhaps largely consisting of mentally ill young men convicted of offences involving various degrees of nuisance and violence. Further, it might be possible that non-offending mentally ill individuals might offend if discharged inappropriately, whilst others who commit 'offences' in hospital, such as assault or indecent exposure, were unlikely to be subject to legal process, but became so on inappropriate discharge. It was here that Dr Bowden's paper was most provocative, because it challenged even this more limited conception of inappropriate placement.

Inappropriate placement

In direct response to Dr Bowden's assertions, the question of whether a substantial number of mentally abnormal offenders were wrongly placed in prison was raised. It was argued that some 1–2% of the sentenced prison population were likely to be psychotic, such that their placement was inappropriate, with the majority of these having a history of psychiatric treatment. If one took an outside figure of 4%, this remained small with respect to the total prison population, but would require an additional 1000 or so secure psychiatric beds; a considerable demand to place on the NHS. However, it was suggested that greater numbers might be involved if it became accepted that psychotic individuals not in an acute phase should be moved to hospital, or if new treatments became available, for instance for some sex offenders. It was further pointed out that Dr Bowden had made it clear that the problem of diversion of the mentally ill from the prisons was not new, and had proved intractable.

Two contributors stated clearly their conviction that whilst it may be essential to improve the provisions for psychiatric treatment within the prison service, the prison system could not be seen as therapeutic in itself. However, it was suggested that, when the chronically mentally ill found themselves in prison, then the prison was part of 'community care' for those who have offended. However, Dr Bowden's apparent suggestion that acutely psychotic individuals might be appropriately placed in the prisons was contested, and particularly in the case of young people, placements should always be the responsibility of the NHS rather than the Home Office.

It was stated that social services staff responsible for hostels are reporting that they are expected to take more violent individuals leaving hospital than previously. Consequently they have become less willing to take those with a record of violence, particularly as psychiatric professionals may be reluctant to furnish staff with relevant information concerning such patients, or to support them in requests for re-admission to hospital. However, evidence from the US was also cited which suggested that patients admitted to psychiatric hospitals were increasingly prone to violence. Overall, it was suggested that psychiatric hospitals might be restricting access to their facilities in a way detrimental to the mentally abnormal offender, a situation which required investigation and was not explicable simply in terms of the demise of authoritarian nursing. Finally, it was pointed out that whatever the difficulties currently facing homeless individuals with psychiatric problems, they themselves consistently resisted the option of a return to hospital.

The careers of mentally disordered offenders

Despite the rejection of the transcarceration hypothesis, a number of contributors identified the need to understand the processes by which mentally disordered offenders come to find themselves inappropriately imprisoned. It was suggested that the law could be arbitrary and in-humane, failing consistently to divert the mentally disordered at the point of entry. Dr Fowles himself emphasized that evidence from those working in the field suggested that changes in police practice may be affecting the future careers of mentally disordered offenders in the criminal justice system (a point which had been made forcibly in the previous discussion). He argued that it was difficult to get a picture of these processes from the experiences of those present, who represented good practice. It was vital to examine the impact of gatekeepers within the criminal justice system, whose effect was to make the consequences of offending haphazard and variable, especially for young offenders. Out-comes are dependent on which police force, CPS branch or prison the mentally disordered individual came into contact with. With respect to the hospital system, it was important to differentiate between those discharged from the hospitals (who leave by the 'back door'), and those who now fail to gain admission to hospital in the first place (for whom the 'front door' has closed). It is vital that we come to understand how mentally disordered offenders come to receive their first probation order or prison sentence, thus enabling improved organization of prior access to psychiatric services, possibly before offending occurs. In general, the rejection of a simple transcarceration hypothesis should not imply that we currently understand or should not be concerned about the processes by which the mentally ill become criminalized.

The planning of future services

Many of the comments already reported bear directly upon questions about the types of services required and the way in which future services should be planned. The concern expressed over the local variations in the ways in which mentally disordered offenders are treated and the general arbitrariness of these processes led Dr Fowles to emphasize that any discussion of quality of life and quality of care should involve some notion of equality of life and care. The problem for the NHS in catering for the small number of those psychotic sentenced inmates inappropriately placed in the prisons has already been identified. It was further argued that providing secure psychiatric hospital places for these individuals required that we study how it is possible to provide care in secure conditions as well. Despite a number of calls for more containment to be available within NHS facilities, it was questioned whether it was feasible for changes that have occurred within hospital practice to be generally reversed; can the locks go back? At the same time, can the special hospitals be successfully reformed?

The need to provide improved services within the prisons was discussed. It was pointed out that, unlike their colleagues in the hospital services, the prison authorities had no choice about who they should take. It was necessary to improve both the general conditions and the hospital services within the prisons. Finally, the need to provide for care within the community, and especially to take into account the needs of less serious offenders was emphasized. In rejecting the Penrose hypothesis, the idea that the only form of care which should be provided for the social deviant is institutional should also be abandoned. Anxieties about transcarceration, and about more complex processes by which the mentally ill may become criminalized, should not result in a return to the old system of large asylums.

7

Defining need and evaluating services

J. K. WING

Introduction

My task is to provide a general introduction to research into ways of defining and measuring the needs of people who are mentally ill and into the efficacy of the various methods that society has used to try to meet those needs. I shall not be concerned with the special needs of mentally ill offenders but the same principles of investigation apply. It is convenient to divide the subject matter into three parts: epidemiology, needs assessment and service evaluation.

Before starting I will specify a particular meaning for three key terms: 'care', care 'agents' and service 'settings'. Understanding the differences between them is basic to clarity of thought about evaluation. 'Care' includes all forms of personal interventions, from medication through counselling to welfare support. 'Agents' are the people, professional and informal, who provide the care. 'Settings' comprise the various structures in which the care is given. All three terms are sometimes characterized as services, so each should be understood as being in quotation marks in what follows, in order to emphasize their differential significance.

The epidemiology of need

An epidemiological perspective is essential for the understanding of any disorder. David Mechanic pointed out, when he first understood what epidemiology meant, that this was what many sociologists thought they had been doing most of their lives.

In that spirit I will quote some figures about crime, produced by a biostatistician, Morton Kramer (1989), for a book about epidemiology (see Table 7.1). They show the number of people, per 100 000 US

Table 7.1. *Number of people, per 100 000 US population, resident in specified types of institution on decennial census days from 1950 to 1980*

Type of institution	1950	1960	1970	1980
Mental institutions	405.5	351.3	213.5	112.7
Homes for aged and dependent	196.1	261.9	456.4	629.7
Correctional institutions	174.8	193.0	161.4	205.9
All other	259.0	246.1	215.3	152.0
Total	1035.4	1052.3	1046.6	1100.3
Total resident population of US (000s)	151 326	179 323	203 302	226 546

Source: Kramer M. (1989).

population, who had been resident in institutions on decennial census days from 1950 to 1980. The overall ratio has remained remarkably steady but the same cannot be said of its components. While that for mental institutions has dropped to about one quarter of the 1950 figure, the ratio for the elderly and dependent has trebled. In 1950, the ratio for mental hospitals was the highest, in 1980 it was lowest, lower than that for prisons.

The interactional dynamics of these groups cannot be determined from such figures (Kramer provides a sophisticated analysis and commentary) but they suggest interesting questions for our own country, which echo those considered in the papers by Drs Fowles and Bowden. A more direct perspective is provided by an index of social deprivation, which can be used to identify geographical areas likely to be of particular concern. A recent publication of results from eight British Psychiatric Case Registers (Wing, 1989*a*) shows the population growth or decline in the local districts during the sixty years from 1921 to 1981. Oxford, for example, doubled its population in this period while that of Camberwell was halved. Medium-sized industrial cities like Cardiff, Nottingham and Southampton stayed approximately at the national level. Worcester and Kidderminster were closer to Oxford while Salford was closer to Camberwell. When the Jarman index of deprivation for the health districts is added, the correspondence between the attractiveness of an area measured in this way and the sociodemographic indices is apparent. It has been shown that some measures of utilization of psychiatric services are correlated with the Jarman index (Hirsch, 1988; Jarman, 1983, 1984).

The 'breeder' hypothesis aside, a two-part explanation may be put forward that attractive areas are acquiring relatively healthy newcomers, while deprived areas not only suffer from the out-migration but some also have an attraction of their own for people who seek for anonymity. There is a danger of over-simplification since the index combines items representing poverty, social isolation, and ethnicity, apart from age and sex.

Not all of these are equally predictive, for example, of admission rates to psychiatric units or of the numbers of residents who have stayed up to five years. It has long been a truism of psychiatric epidemiology that indices of social isolation are particularly useful in identifying vulnerable areas.

The relevance for evaluating programmes of mental health care is obvious: the results found in one area can only be generalized for planning purposes in another after exercising extreme caution about the relevant sociodemographic differences. A more specific example is the new mental health service provided in the Worcester Development Project before the large hospital at Powick was closed early in 1989 (Wing, 1990*a*). The service was set up as a model and does indeed excel, for example, in terms of places in purpose built day units. But it is clear that conclusions about the success of hospital closure there cannot readily be transferred to Salford or Camberwell.

Needs assessment

The concept of need draws upon all the disparate elements of evaluative research and provides the link between problem, action and evaluation. The most common criticism of the concept is that it fails to distinguish between statements of fact and statements of value. But this itself is the central problem in any application of research results. Since it is impossible to leave value out, it is best to arrange for the presence of value to be clearly visible.

I use Graham Matthew's definitions of the basic terms 'need', 'demand' and 'utilization' because they are so clear and economical and the principles behind them are sound (Matthew, 1971):

A need for medical care exists when an individual has an illness or disability for which there is effective and acceptable treatment or care. It can be defined either in terms of the type of illness or disability causing the need or of the treatment or facilities for treatment required to meet it. A demand for care exists when an individual considers that he has a need and wishes to receive care. Utilization occurs when an individual actually receives care. Need is not necessarily expressed as demand and demand is not necessarily followed by utilization, while, on the other hand, there can be demand and utilization without real underlying need for the particular service used.

(*ibid*)

These definitions apply specifically to medical diagnosis and treatment. Their content must be broadened when applied to psychiatric and social problems. For our purposes it is better to begin with the concept of social disablement. I suspect we should all be on common ground if the most fundamental aim in relation to mental illness were stated to be to prevent or minimize social disablement by dealing with its major components – disease, disability, disadvantage and demoralization or distress. Each of these can be measured with a fair degree of reliability; certainly enough to make useful research feasible (Wing, 1989*b*; 1990*b*).

Most evaluations using a concept of need have been made in global terms, with one or more clinicians or research workers in effect making private judgements as to the kinds of care and service thought to be necessary and then recording whether of not they had been provided. Detailed measurements of clinical and social problems are often provided, and make for a degree of repeatability between studies, but the paths from these problems to the action regarded as appropriate are not publicly specified.

In order to convince planners and administrators that the results have reasonable solidity and meaning, it is necessary to make the whole process of needs assessment more transparent and also to add the dimension of cost. Values then really do come to the surface and begin to compete with each other.

What, therefore, has to be done is to set standards for expected levels of functioning, list the actions that current professional practice regards as appropriate in the case of deviation from each of the standards, and provide rules for deciding whether the action has or has not been taken. This provides a basis for prescribing action to meet the needs that are identified but not met. The process of assessment is then repeated as often as necessary in order to test the assumptions made in the preceding assessments and to minimize the level of unmet need. Such a procedure has several advantages:

(*a*) It is firmly based in current professional practice and, indeed, can be seen as a public expression of it.
(*b*) It ensures that all methods of 'care', professional and informal 'agents' who provide the care, and service 'settings' in which the

Table 7.2. *Areas of functioning that might be problematic (each to be rated present or absent)*

Clinical problems	Personal and social problems
Psychotic symptoms	Self care
Depression	Household skills, shopping
Anxiety	Occupational skills
Obsessions	Social interaction skills
Negative symptoms	Basic literacy and numeracy
Cognitive deficits	Money management
Distress	Decision making and personal responsibility
Disturbed behaviour	Family problems
Alcohol and drug misuse	Use of local amenities – public transport, cafes, etc.
Eating disorders	
Somatoform disorders	

Note: Other factors affecting the manifestation of problems should also be noted, e.g. local topography, isolation, poverty, employment levels, housing, recreational facilities, crime.

agents operate, are considered as options, not only those that are actually available.

(c) It diminishes subjectivity and therefore increases comparability.

(d) If applied across a sufficiently representative group of individuals with mental health problems it can provide an estimate of the needs for service 'settings' and for their staffing, as well as for types of 'care'.

(e) All the assumptions involved can be scrutinized and challenged.

Tables 7.2–7.4 provide an outline of the assessment procedure, the decision points, and the areas of functioning covered (Brewin *et al.*, 1987; Brewin & Wing, 1988). They can be adapted for use with other groups than the one we studied.

The system has been created for research purposes. If used more routinely, in simplified form, there would be a less meticulous attention to detail and more reliance on the need for staff and settings that were already in place, since that would be its major function. The costs of items of care could also be calculated. However, the system could also be used for local operational research into gaps in services. Independently minded professionals, both clinical and managerial, would wish to have that kind of information for planning purposes.

Table 7.3. *List of possible interventions available for those rated as
having a problem related to 'active
psychotic symptoms'*

Prescription of correct medication
Supervision of medication
Coping advice to patient
Coping advice to relatives
Family intervention
Sheltered accommodation
Support and reassurance

For each intervention, consider whether:

There is a need for it:
If so, is it:
– met?
– unmet?
– likely to be needed in the future?

If no need for it:
– is there overprovision?

Table 7.4. *Audit of care provided*

Provide the recommended item of care for each unmet need
Follow up and repeat needs assessment
Discover whether needs are now met
If not, why not?
Are new interventions necessary?
Are there new needs?
Continue to follow up as above

Audit of services provided

For each intervention (for a single patient), choose:

minimal service agent, e.g. befriender, CPN, social worker, psychologist, etc.
minimal service setting, e.g. office, home visit, day centre, etc.

For each set of interventions (for single patient), choose:

agent(s) and setting(s) likely to meet needs

For each group of individuals, consider the ideal arrangement of agents and
settings that would most effectively and economically cater for the needs of the
group

Match these against what is currently available

Consider the policy indications

Evaluating services

This brief review of two basic requirements – an epidemiological base and a sure grasp of technical measurement – illustrates nevertheless the weakness of a general approach to evaluation. It can only be discussed with proper meaning in relation to a problem. Once that is specified, the details of designing a research project intended to provide an answer can begin to be tackled. No design, no method of sampling and no set of measurements will suit all problems.

Psychiatric epidemiology has a long history and, accepting David Mechanic's argument that much sociological survey research must be included under this heading, there have been some distinguished examples in the field of criminology. I am not so sure that there is yet much of an epidemiological perspective to the evaluation of services, if I can expand the meaning of the word to include correctional establishments. For example, what clinical, personal, family or social difference does it make if someone with schizophrenia who commits a minor offence spends the next six months in a prison, or in a special hostel, or in hospital, or at home?

Obviously the constraints of sentencing, to say nothing of the sampling problems, rule out controlled studies. But very few controlled studies have been carried out even in the absence of such constraints.

Naturalistic designs are more flexible and highly adaptable to circumstances, but the less rigorous the design the more caution must be exercised when interpreting the results. In the case of the social psychiatry unit of the Medical Research Council, studies have ranged from action research, with studies of homeless men sleeping under the arches, which reached quite specific conclusions without being much acted upon (Leach & Wing, 1980; Tidmarsh & Wood, 1972), through tighter investigations of 'settings' such as sheltered workshops, day hospitals and day centres, hostels, and group homes (Wing & Hailey, 1972; Wing & Olsen, 1979), to larger-scale comparative projects (Brown *et al.*, 1966; Wing, 1982; Wing & Bennett, 1989; Wing & Brown, 1970).

Out of this range of projects, those based directly or indirectly on the Camberwell Register and on close interactions between clinicians, administrators and research workers during the late 1960s, have perhaps had the most evident practical consequences (Wing & Hailey, 1972). Most of the recommendations made have actually been put into practice.

Of our current work, I would particularly commend a study that started in the MRC social psychiatry unit in 1980 and still has a year or so to run in

Table 7.5. *Rundown to closure of Darenth Park Hospital – first phase*

Place at follow-up	Clinical group			Total
	'Aloof'	'Passive'	'Sociable'	
Movers				
Another hospital	26 (5)	10 (2)	44 (7)	80 (14)
Hostel, etc.	8 (—)	30 (—)	161 (6)	199 (6)
Stayers				
In Darenth	182 (31)	94 (11)	338 (63)	614 (105)
Total	216 (36)	134 (13)	543 (76)	893 (125)

Note: Figures in parentheses are number of deaths.
Source: Wing L, 1989.

the successor unit. It is concerned with the run down to closure of a hospital for the mentally handicapped. The hospital had already been running down for many years and most of the residents remaining were severely handicapped. A matched-control succeeded by self-control design was adopted. During the first five years of the project, residents were moved out of hospital to whatever apparently suitable alternative accommodation could be found.

The results of research on the first phase have now been published by Lorna Wing (1989). They make compelling reading for anyone who is interested in objective analysis and comment. Because the problems of sampling are somewhat less complicated than those posed by long-term mental illness, a map of the issues posed in undertaking such crucial tests of current policies is very clearly laid out before the reader. Tables 7.5 and 7.6 provide a very brief summary. The three clinical groups shown in the Table 7.5 are differentiated on the basis of a reliable procedure for collecting information on the developmental history and current handicaps, behaviour and skills, and represent degrees of severity of social impairment. Other groupings (in particular, physical handicap) are also used in analysis. Most of the movers were placed into 'community' accommodation that was already available, including for example another but smaller hospital. Less disabled people were, of course, likely to leave first.

During the second phase, which ended with the closure of the hospital in August 1988, new purpose-built accommodation was provided. The results of the second stage research will soon be available. Julian Leff's

Table 7.6. *Rundown to closure of Darenth Park Hospital – summary of changes*

Summary of changes in the movers	
Skills – no change	Privacy, use of community services – increased for passive and social groups of movers
Behaviour – no change	Education, occupation, leisure activities – decreased for social group
Life style – no change	

Summary of changes in matched stayers
Initial status virtually identical to those of the movers
At follow-up, no change

Source: Wing L, 1989.

studies at Friern and Claybury, using a similar design, are likely to have the same impact on the mental health services if they can be carried through over the same period of time.

This paper is not chiefly about implementation and I will only suggest that the motivation for undertaking evaluative research should be maintained through scientific curiosity. If the results do sometimes get translated into action (even if indirectly, after long delay and without any understanding of where the ideas come from), that is a bonus. But although the examples of evaluative research (research into destitution excepted) that I have given are at some distance from the topic of this meeting, I hope it is clear that somewhat similar problems of design, sampling and measurement have had to be overcome and that the practical consequences and implications have by no means been negligible.

Discussion

The discussion focused on the inherent difficulties encountered in attempting to provide independent and objective measures of patients' needs, the relation between these measures of need and the evaluation of patient services, and the significance of such data for the effective provision of care.

The evaluation of needs: patient and provider perceptions

It was emphasized that the experienced, or felt, needs of patients should be acknowledged, as distinct from patient needs as defined by health care professionals. The view that patients' perceptions can simply be measured when they 'vote with their feet' was criticized: ways had to be found to investigate and champion actively the needs of mentally disordered offenders. Professor Wing accepted that the issue of who defines need was basic. However, patients' perceptions, and those of their relatives, were not always based on adequate information concerning treatment options: consultation without input from informed professionals was meaningless. As a result, patients tended to wish to remain in institutions with which they were familiar. It was especially important to speak for patients with severe mental disability. It was suggested that citizen advocates could bridge the gap between the perceptions of patients and the preconceptions of professionals, but citizen advocates also had their own preconceptions.

It was suggested that a clear distinction between patients' needs and the ways in which these might be met should be maintained. In some areas there might be professional unanimity on the best responses to particular needs, but in the case of mentally disordered offenders this was not so; everyone thought they should be treated 'somewhere else'. Professor Wing took up this point and warned against reifying assessments of need into practical recommendations. By clarifying issues of need, one often did not resolve issues of provision, but raised the temperature of debates surrounding them, although these could now be conducted more rationally, with opposing ideas having to compete against one another.

Doubt was raised about the possibility of evaluating needs completely independently from the types of social and psychiatric intervention which professionals were able to provide. It was argued that need assessments by researchers were structured by conventional expectations of available care. Further, the clear explication of value judgments associated with particular pieces of research was no guard against other value judgments being smuggled into needs evaluations. It was suggested that the contamination of need categories by available treatment categories might be particularly problematic in the case of mentally disordered offenders, whose view of their needs was liable to be very different from that of professional researchers and practitioners. Professor Wing argued that the best way to deal with these issues was for competition between different professional approaches to occur within an academic debate, so that detached research could be distinguished from that of over-committed product champions.

Another contributor re-emphasized the need to foster truly independent research. Reference was made to Coid's studies, which indicated that diagnoses may sometimes be changed so as to fit people with particular facilities (Coid, 1988*a*,*b*). There was a need for high-quality research, because professionals were being increasingly encouraged to take account of provision in their assessments, with the prospect that clinical judgments might become resource-led (Griffiths, 1988). A question was raised about whether the research of Professor Wing and others could be put to use in the current political climate. NHS managers wanted to know if there was a viable market for particular services, i.e. if they would generate income. Could this approach co-exist with that of needs assessment? Professor Wing suggested that research should come from institutions of a high standard, primarily universities. By making research information available, it was possible to compare various types of provision. Currently, judgments were made on poor information. The possibility of more open and thus better justified service judgments was consistent with the White Paper's insistence on clinical audit (Department of Health, 1989*a*).

The evaluation of treatment services

One contributor identified two questions raised by the paper; how should the success of a service be defined, and how can this be measured against the investment of resources in the service? Professor Wing argued that the possibility of measuring success was built into the assessment procedures. By measuring and then re-measuring needs, one could assess whether relevant interventions were available or not. Furthermore, these assessments could be open to public view. He referred to research in his own region, which had shown gaps in the provision of community facilities through needs assessment studies. Although decisions to provide services had to be made 'top down', they could be based on information concerning the needs of patients, rather than information concerning the operational problems of the existing health care system. However, it was pointed out that the day-to-day business of health service management primarily involved choosing between particular policies or developments. Professor Wing responded by accepting that the manager's task was primarily to choose between competing priorities, but this choice could be informed by assessments of need. It was also argued that this information could be relevant to the evaluation of unmet needs experienced by the mentally disordered from minority ethnic groups, either directly as a result of racism, or through social disadvantages experienced more generally but loaded on to particular ethnic communities.

It was argued that, along with the needs of clients, the associated needs of service providers to assess rapidly whether particular policies were working should be considered. During periods of service transition management problems were liable to occur, and the rapid gathering and use of information at these times was difficult. However, the advent of micro-computer systems allowed for far more rapid evaluation of complex information, based upon clinicians collecting their own data. Further, micro-computers can be linked to develop such possibilities. The ethical problems concerning the storage of data about patients on micro-computer systems were raised, although these were not thought to invalidate the clinical possibilities of the new technology. One contributor argued that a presentation he had witnessed of this sort of data suggested that the process was too laborious, and required too many people to collect it. Professor Wing drew a distinction between complex independent research methods, and 'cut down' systems which were suitable for use by clinical teams, and relied on the collection and presentation of simple information.

8

Black people, mental health and the criminal justice system[1]

D. BROWNE, E. FRANCIS and I. CROWE

Introduction

There is ample evidence in the psychiatric literature to show that black people are over-represented as patients in psychiatric hospitals.[2] Over the past two decades there has been a steady increase in the reported levels of admissions of black people to psychiatric hospitals (Cochrane, 1971; Bebbington et al., 1981; Harrison et al., 1988). Epidemiological studies show that most of these hospital admissions are accompanied by a diagnosis of a major psychotic illness, particularly schizophrenia. Earlier researchers suggested that nativity was the pre-eminent factor in determining risk of hospital admission partly because of hypotheses that mental illness was a consequence of migration (Bagley, 1976). More recent studies, however, claim that ethnicity (regardless of place of birth) is the crucial variable (Burke, 1984).

Some of the more recent findings have aroused considerable debate in both academic and professional circles and in the black community. There has been little agreement or consistency amongst academics as to a singular or multiple cause for the over-representation, and speculation has ranged from genetic susceptibility, adverse reactions to racism and cultural differences between psychiatrist and patient. However, the professional consensus is that there is an ethnic 'vulnerability' to mental illness somewhat separate from the quality of professional practice (diagnosis and treatment) or institutional processes (compulsory admission) (Littlewood, 1981; Littlewood & Lipsedge, 1981). The challenge, then, is to arrive at an explanation that would interrogate these speculations. It is most notable that the idea that hospital admissions may not be a true reflection of levels of mental illness in the black community (or that referral of black people to psychiatric hospitals is subject to different criteria) has not been given rigorous scrutiny.

We will try to show in this paper that black people are more likely than their white counterparts to come to the attention of psychiatrists, regardless of their presenting symptoms. In addition, we also argue that the disproportionate number of black people in psychiatric facilities is also dependent upon different clinical criteria, e.g. dangerousness, severity of illness, and prognosis. Finally, we also suggest that the experience prior to the clinical encounter may be central in determining whether a black person sees a psychiatrist at all. Therefore, contacts with social services, physicians, health care and law enforcement agencies may be important in averting or precipitating psychological crises.

Empirical work in progress by the authors has been guided by the following process model (Fig. 8.1) which serves as a means of understanding the stages in the antecedents to black people's contact with psychiatrists.

There is empirical evidence to support each stage within this model which could be unified by a theory based on the concept of 'deviance' (Donzelot, 1979). What may otherwise appear to be discrete processes affecting the individual in relation to just one agency (psychiatry) could alternatively be analysed as a circuitous process involving a number of agencies which apply labels of abnormality and have the power to exercise coercion and incarceration. It is evident from official statistics

General population

Increased recognition/surveillance of black people
(Social service, mental illness and crime)

Increased risk of emergency psychiatric referrals
by multiple agencies
(Police, GPs, social workers, courts, prisons)

Psychiatric assessment more likely to lead
to hospital admission.

Fig. 8.1. Antecedents to contacts between black people and psychiatric services.

that the social antecedents of black mentally abnormal offenders could be traced back to the diagnosis of educational subnormality and behavioural disorder in black children by the Schools Psychological Service (Bagley, 1976; Coard, 1977; ILEA, 1981, 1985).

Furthermore, social service practices could be examined. Black people are traditionally more likely than their white counterparts to be in crises or emergency circumstances leading to contacts with welfare agencies (Ahmed *et al.*, 1986). The crisis intervention work by these agencies often takes the place of sustained, long-term or preventative support and it is likely that decision-making by these agencies in a substantial proportion of cases may be wholly inappropriate and could directly lead to referrals to psychiatry in general or forensic services in particular.

This argument is supported by research findings (Hitch & Clegg, 1980) which showed that the circumstances surrounding hospital admission differed for 'New Commonwealth-born' and 'native-born' patients. Across all psychiatric hospital admissions, black patients are three to four times more likely to be admitted with the involvement of police. Other studies have shown a similar preponderance of police involvement in hospital admissions and the relative absence of GPs in this process in relation to ethnicity (Rwegellera, 1977; Littlewood & Lipsedge, 1981; Harrison *et al.*, 1988). It is this pattern of diagnosis of severe mental disorder in Afro-Caribbean patients, along with emergency assessment, involvement of a number of agencies apart from mental health workers and the use of procedures under the Mental Health Act 1983 which has a direct bearing upon referrals to forensic psychiatry. Our point of departure in this paper is the initial assessment in the magistrates' court setting.

Outline of research

There is very little research material which specifically examines the role of the criminal justice system as a factor in the psychiatric treatment of Afro-Caribbean people. By the criminal justice system we refer, of course, to the police, courts and prison institutions which have the power to exercise a certain latitude in enforcing and interpreting the law for or against the interests of certain sections of the community, whether by conscious strategy (institutional racism) or by unconscious racism or prejudices.

Work has been previously conducted by MIND which clearly illustrates that Afro-Caribbean people are considerably more likely than their white counterparts to be detained by police under s.136 of the Mental

Health Act 1983 and taken to a place of safety (Rogers & Faulkner, 1987). However, this research does not pursue the antecedents or consequences of this process in terms of Mental Health Act procedures in the courts or their relation to criminal justice processes. There are considerably more concerns for the black experience of psychiatry.

Black people are over-represented amongst those coming before the courts; amongst those who receive custodial sentences (NACRO, 1985); and in the prisons and young offender institutions (Home Office, 1988*b*). It seems almost axiomatic that there should also be an over-representation amongst prisoners on psychiatric remand and in the category of offenders who receive hospital orders.

Funding from the Commission for Racial Equality presented an opportunity to begin to address some of these concerns. However, the funding was limited and it was decided to undertake a study that would be essentially exploratory in nature. The purpose of the study was two-fold: first, to clarify the hypotheses that it would be useful to test more adequately in a fuller study; second, to explore some of the practical and methodological problems likely to be encountered. The study was therefore seen as essentially a prelude to further work, rather than as producing conclusive findings. This precluded the collection of data on a large scale, and it was decided to adopt a 'case study' approach, where the case was a particular locality, the features of which could be studied in some detail. A particular inner city area was chosen. It had a sizeable black population (in the two boroughs involved, black people constituted 15% and 20% of the populations), was well served by psychiatric facilities, including a psychiatric teaching hospital, had a local magistrates' court close by and a male remand prison in the vicinity. Hence it promised reasonable access to the necessary sources of information. As with any such study, the limited generalizability of the data must be acknowledged.

The research was based on identifying key decision-making points within the process for study. This is derived, in this instance, from the model adopted by Coid (1987) and as indicated the point chosen for study was the remand decision (see Fig. 8.2).

All cases recorded as remanded for psychiatric reports during 1987 were extracted from the register at the magistrates' court. Information was then obtained on these cases from the court register and files from the nearby psychiatric hospital, from the male remand prison and from the probation service. In addition, interviews were undertaken with a small number of professionals involved in decision-making; magistrates, court

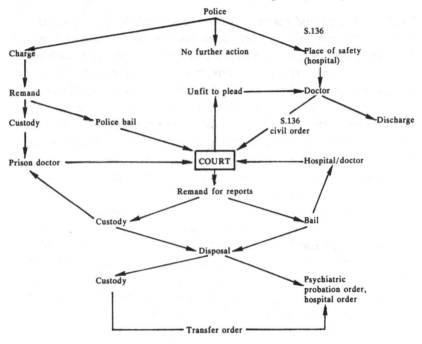

Fig. 8.2. Mentally disordered offenders: a decision-making framework.

clerks, probation officers, and psychiatrists. Surveys were also under-taken of local solicitors' firms and local community agencies providing services likely to be used by those needing psychiatric help.

A project steering group was convened consisting of workers from the police, probation service, prisons, psychiatry and community groups. The project was organized by the National Association of the Care and Resettlement of Offenders (NACRO) in collaboration with the Afro-Caribbean Mental Health Association and was funded by the Commission for Racial Equality. The research aimed to examine these issues:

(i)   the extent to which black people are remanded for psychiatric reports by magistrates' courts;
(ii) the nature of the remands;
(iii) the service provisions for this client group in the community.

Research findings

Some principal issues, though not the main point of interest here, may be briefly itemized:

(*a*) As anticipated, the lack of routine ethnic monitoring in all agencies, bar the prison, made it difficult to classify by race.

(*b*) The variety of ways in which psychiatric reports come to be presented to the court, made it difficult to extract a satisfactory sample through court records. In particular, 'private' psychiatric reports are often arranged by defence lawyers, and these do not necessarily show up in the court records.

(*c*) Having extracted a case, it is often quite difficult to follow that case through the medical and penal systems to get adequate information.

(*d*) Because one is dealing with infrequent events, a large amount of effort is necessary to obtain even quite modest numbers, thus limiting the kinds of analysis and conclusions that are possible.

The defendants

Of 38 000 cases heard at an Inner London Magistrates' Court during 1987, 70 were extracted as having been remanded for psychiatric assessment. This was almost certainly an under-representation of the full number of cases in which psychiatric assessments were produced (see (ii) above). The sample comprised 38% white defendants while 33% were black (Afro-Caribbean). Asians comprised 3%. The ethnicity of 26% was unknown. Of the 52 sample members who were racially identifiable it can be seen that almost half were black or Asian. Whilst acknowledging the smallness of the sample this is clearly a marked over-representation of ethnic minorities, and Afro-Caribbean people in particular.

A number of factors were examined to see whether they had any relevance to the likelihood of psychiatric remand and may be briefly summarized:

(*a*) Gender and age – The sample was predominantly young and male, in keeping with the normal workload of courts.

(*b*) Previous convictions – Almost half the sample had no, or only one, previous convictions (49%). A higher proportion of black than white defendants remanded for reports had two or more previous convictions.

(*c*) Previous psychiatric contact – A higher number of black defendants had had previous contact with psychiatric services (26%). This concurs with research findings in relation to higher hospital admissions of black people. Discussions with magistrates and solicitors did not suggest that previous psychiatric contact on the part of the defendant would mean necessarily that a psychiatric report would be requested, but certainly there appeared to be more of a connection with regard to the black cohort.

(*d*) Current offence – Black defendants were more likely than white defendants to have been involved in what may be termed 'personal' rather than property offences.[3]

(*e*) Bail or custody – Of the black sample 45% was likely to be remanded in custody compared with 39% of the whites. Parallels can be drawn with the experiences of black people generally within the criminal justice system. Most notably, the black defendants were granted bail in markedly fewer cases (14%) compared with 48% for their white counterparts. This finding is in keeping with the existing data illustrating that black defendants are generally less likely to receive bail for criminal offences. Only three people in the whole sample were remanded on a s.35 hospital order.

We would conjecture that the criteria on which bail applications are based are related to subjective notions of dangerousness and public menace which bears little relation to objective measures of safety and risk. A complex interplay of forces appears to be at work here. First, there is a traditional and much documented problem associated with the quality of decision-making in the criminal justice system and the latitude allowed to law enforcement agencies to label certain forms of deviancy as either medical or criminal or both (Prins, 1980; Brooks, 1984). Secondly, stereotypes of black people which generally exist in the society can be combined with notions of pathological danger producing an increased tariff of risk (Whitehouse, 1983). Thirdly, these notions are combined to produce a procedure for sentencing and disposal which consistently prefers to err on the side of caution. Given these factors, and the stereotypes which exist in relation to mental illness in general, it is not surprising that the treatment of black mentally disordered offenders should be consistently associated with coercion and containment. This is illustrated in an under-representation of black people in nonpsychiatric probation orders and an over-representation in cases where treatment is attached to probation orders. We would also suggest that this is based on assessments of danger as opposed to the welfare of the 'offender'.

(*f*) Length of remand – About half of all remands were no more than four weeks duration, but the remainder were spread over quite a long period (24 weeks in one instance).

(g) Disposals – About a third of all disposals (36%) involved an order (hospital or probation with psychiatric conditions) rather than a sentence. Black offenders were particularly likely to receive a psychiatric probation order (43%).

(h) Diagnosis – These were extremely diverse, but black remandees were almost twice as likely to be assessed as suffering from some form of serious mental illness such as schizophrenia.

The professionals

It is not possible to describe in detail the material obtained from the various professional groups involved in the psychiatric remand process, and therefore what is said will be confined to three points of interest that emerged. The first point centres round the problem of identifying the appropriateness of invoking a psychiatric dimension in a case. There was variation in what magistrates saw as the purpose of a psychiatric remand. The nature of the offence alone was not a determining factor. What emerged was that the decision whether to remand is essentially an intuitive decision. Such subjective assessments may well permit prejudicial and discriminatory practices to develop. It was also noticeable that the (admittedly few) magistrates had only a limited awareness of the provisions of s.35–38 of the Mental Health Act 1983.

Another aspect of this concern about the appropriateness of psychiatric referral was highlighted when talking to probation officers and solicitors. Invoking the possibility of psychiatric assistance was seen as a way of getting a more sympathetic response to a client and possibly a more 'lenient' disposal. However, this may not be necessarily something that benefits a client if, as indicated above, it leads to a high chance of remand in custody. On the other hand, a failure to recognize the possible psychiatric dimension of a case can have tragic consequences. In one case cited by a solicitor, a disturbed young woman committed suicide after being released on bail, and in another case a man who failed to receive treatment for progressive schizophrenia later committed manslaughter. There is thus a danger of both false positives and false negatives. The question therefore arises whether there should be clearer guidelines regarding the purpose of psychiatric remands and the procedures to be followed in ordering psychiatric reports.

The second point that emerged from talking to the professional groups was the level of concern about the inadequacies of present arrangements for obtaining psychiatric reports, and, in particular, the length of time it often took to obtain reports. This was mentioned by magistrates, clerks, probation officers and solicitors. One consequence of this was what appeared to be the emergence of an informal network and independent initiatives for getting reports done. As has been mentioned, solicitors often arranged for 'private' psychiatric reports. It was mentioned that, amongst the reasons for doing this were that the solicitor could then exercise more control over obtaining the report and the choice of psychiatrist. Probation officers similarly tended to develop contacts with individual psychiatrists. The development of these informal networks and the resort to 'private' reports have considerable implications. In the first place, it is clear that one is not just concerned with medical and judicial issues. The dissatisfaction with present formal arrangements raises questions about the resources and administrative efficiency of the system, and therefore about management issues. There is also a political dimension: in the present climate should an increasing resort to 'private' psychiatric reports be encouraged? A second consideration in relation to the development of informal networks is that, under present conditions, they will tend to be white dominated, and this would work against the interests of black defendants. Whilst the development of good links between the different professional groups may be desirable, it is perhaps important that it should happen in a structured way, through inter-agency working groups, rather than in an *ad hoc* fashion.

The third and final point to emerge from interviews with professionals was a dissatisfaction with the Prison Medical Service. This was expressed in terms of both the level of treatment available within prison and what was generally felt to be the poorer quality of psychiatric reports provided. Magistrates interviewed felt that reports from the prison did not contain sufficient information and tended to be concerned solely with fitness to plead rather than with the value of potential disposals. Some NHS psychiatrists were also critical of the quality of reports provided by the Prison Medical Service. A number of options may be possible, including reducing the incidence of remand in custody, but it would also seem to be desirable that prison medical staff should be involved in any inter-agency groups.

The community

Questionnaires were sent to 116, largely voluntary, agencies in the research area. Thirty usable responses were received. (Further work is being pursued on this aspect of the study.) Of these 30, 14 were from agencies offering some form of service specifically for the mentally disordered and black people constituted more than a quarter of the client group in eight of these. The only agency which frequently received referrals from the police had the highest proportion of black clients (40%). Sixteen of the 30 agencies offered a range of services, and did not cater specifically for the mentally disturbed. These had a much lower take up of services by black clients. Although it is not possible to discuss the results in detail, some significant points are raised by this preliminary enquiry into community based provision which require further investigation. In the first place it was noticeable that very few such agencies maintain monitoring systems which enable them to give a good account of their work. Second, the indications were that black people were having to rely on a relatively small number of agencies because these were the only ones prepared and equipped to cater for them; most agencies simply did not offer a service that appealed to black people in need of psychiatric help. Finally there were indications that, due to a lack of assistance or referral at an early stage, black clients were more likely to have to reach a crisis requiring hospitalization before action was taken. Help at an earlier stage might have avoided this.

Conclusion

We have shown that there is a continuity between the treatment of black patients in the mental health services and the processing of black defendants in the criminal justice system. We suggest that the welfare antecedents of black defendants can be traced to prior contacts with multiple agencies ranging from school, social services to primary health care. Experience gained from working in the Legal Advice Unit at the Afro-Caribbean Mental Health Association, which offers legal representation to the black mentally ill, testifies to the double-edged nature of forensic psychiatry, sentencing policy and Mental Health Act procedures. On the one hand, the overwhelming majority of clients who use this service are black people who have been diagnosed as having some mental health problem but who have been charged with criminal offences following public incidents of deviant behaviour. On the other hand, a smaller number of clients who have consciously committed offences have been wrongly diagnosed as mentally ill. In our view this experience points to a system which is in serious dysfunction as the result of inadequate facilities and unclear procedures.

The above findings, though limited by the scope of the research project, lead us to conclude that some of the criteria on which these decisions are based, may be subjective and prejudicial and may lead magistrates to order a greater number of custodial sentences (hospital orders) or psychiatric supervision under probation orders where black people are concerned.

Despite the limited scope of the study that was undertaken, we believe that there is ample information about the experience of the mentally abnormal offender in general and the black defendant in particular that would support a major reform of procedures in the criminal justice system. In particular, we call for the following:

(i)   Greater quality in the assessment of black defendant.
(ii)   More effective monitoring of the processing of black defendants.
(iii)   More consistent criteria for granting of bail and probation orders.
(iv)   Greater consistency in sentencing to ensure that disposals to the prisons or hospitals are both appropriate and in accord with the needs of the defendant/patient.
(v)   More community options for black offender/patients including a greater use of bail hostels accompanied by more appropriate admission criteria.
(vi)   The provision of training for workers in the criminal justice system in the assessment and management of offender/patients.
(vii)   The adoption and implementation of equal opportunities policies and anti-racist action plans by all agencies.
(viii)   The development of routine ethnic monitoring in all agencies so that the adequacy of provision can be investigated.

We would conclude that there is a great need for further research in this area. There is a need for information on the social antecedents of the black defendant and the impact that this may have in determining contact with forensic psychiatry. We were unable to assess the impact of psychiatric history on disposal or the relationship to particular types of offences. Unfortunately, the limitation of the sample did not allow for the inclusion of a representative female group nor indeed the breakdown of the black category which was formulated in accordance with Home Office guidelines.

In light of the fact that there is a dearth of research in the area of black mentally ill offenders generally, there is an even greater need to focus on the experiences of black women who have traditionally been excluded from academic research on race, criminality and psychiatry. A survey conducted by the former GLC Women's Committee highlighted the disproportionate number of black women in Holloway Prison who were inappropriately prescribed psychotropic drugs for reasons of control (Women's Equality Group/LSPU, 1985).

These concerns point to a need for a more thoroughly integrated approach to research in the area of race and criminal justice. Too many studies have concentrated on the number of black people involved in various aspects of the system but there needs to be more research which concentrates on process and the inter-connection between various agencies. It is essential that this work looks at the black experience in terms of gender and social class.

Discussion

The discussion revolved around the issue of ethnic monitoring, but embraced a number of related themes including: problems associated with the monitoring itself, differential responses by treatment agencies, and the modification of racist attitudes.

Problems with ethnic monitoring

The discussion began by focusing on the problem of initiating a programme of ethnic monitoring within a care agency. Particular reference was made to the way in which the issue was currently being handled within the probation service. Here, the problem was one of which categories to employ in the new system. This was despite the overall enthusiasm of the service for the general principle of monitoring. It was argued, in response, that there were standard classifications, so this was not ultimately a practical problem. The key issue was how the monitoring was to be used. It was not intended to investigate the points at which particular disadvantages became built into the lives of individuals. It could relate to family circumstances and cultural questions and to the response of agencies. It was claimed that nobody was ready to talk about policy development unless the effects of policies could be actually measured. The prison service and the courts had begun to embrace ethnic monitoring. Probation officers may be afraid of the potential misuse of the information, but safeguards could be found.

One contributor asked whether ethnic monitoring was used in the special hospitals, either by the Home Office (in relation to patients on restriction orders) or the Special Hospitals Service Authority. The over-representation of black people on hospital orders (s.37 *Mental Health Act*, 1983) was acknowledged. The problems associated with ethnic monitoring by police forces were also mentioned. How far should such monitoring go? Should it include motoring offences, for instance. The difficulty in assessing without ethnic monitoring the possible racist bias in the use of s.136 of the *Mental Health Act* 1983 was identified. The interest of psychiatrists in ethnic monitoring was also reported, but it was pointed out that the data which those in the medical profession were required to collect, the 'Korner data', specifically excluded reference to ethnicity. It was difficult to see how the two systems could be reconciled.

Iain Crowe supported the use of the Commission for Racial Equality guidelines, but pointed out that monitoring could be both used and abused; social enquiry reports were specifically meant not to refer to subjects' ethnicity, but ethnic monitoring of outcomes was still required.

Inequalities in the provision of treatment advice

Mr Francis suggested that the problems surrounding ethnic monitoring arose because the monitoring was not sophisticated enough. It was not sufficient to know how many people used a particular service. It was important to know about the quality of the service they received, and about the ways in which they moved through the service, information which could be used in conjunction with measures of need. There was a need for a wider conception of ethnic monitoring. Black people had special difficulties, but so did other groups. The development of new community care arrangements provided an ideal opportunity for a development of monitoring procedures, but this would not happen if black people were thought of as a marginal group whose needs were radically different from others in society. In the end, everyone wanted similar things: housing, employment, and a decent choice between kinds of care, both in custodial and community settings.

It was argued that monitoring should embrace broad processes of decision-making; it was difficult to piece together the differences between the careers of white and black individuals from local studies. However, these were disturbing in themselves. More black people were stopped and searched, they were less likely to receive a police caution, they were less likely to be sentenced by the courts once tried, but were still over-represented in the sentenced population. All this gave an indication of the places to examine when studying different careers. The issues remained complex; for instance, young blacks were less likely to admit offences so they were less likely to receive cautions. There was a need to look in detail at what happened to them. Although attenders at conferences say they do not know what is happening, they do know where to look! There was a need for more funds to be committed to research in the area.

The ways in which decisions were made to direct people to special services required examination. Knowledge was needed about how people were channelled through services. It was argued that problems could arise when there were too many specialized care agencies, such as those for ethnic minorities; they were needed to help people but they could become ways in which particular groups were marginalized. This occurred at the 'stress points'. Special alternatives to custody were needed, but these had to be set up in such a way as to place the onus on existing services to change their patterns of practice in concert with the specialist agency. Procedures had to be changed throughout the system, rather than relying on specialized agencies which allowed others to divest themselves of their responsibilities. Reference was made to Dr Joseph's psychiatric liaison scheme at Bow Street Magistrates' Court, which seemed to work well in counteracting this effect. Special agencies for the ethnic minorities were required to alleviate the misery individuals were currently experiencing because institutions took a long time to change, but it should not be assumed that the problem was solved because a special agency had been set up. It was further argued that specialist agencies could set precedents in the development of better practices. However, it was also noted that it was asking a great deal of the specialist agencies for the ethnic minorities to take on the dual role of supporting disadvantaged individuals and initiating better practices, particularly when the agencies also receive many requests from other organizations trying to divest themselves of their responsibilities.

There was a discussion of the role of the Home Office in decisions affecting mentally disordered offenders from ethnic minority groups. It was pointed out that the Home Office consumed, but did not provide, psychiatric services; however, the Home Office was responsible for decisions concerning restriction orders under the *Mental Health Act* 1983. The Home Office needed to monitor and to explain its decisions to clients who often could not understand them. Responsible medical officers claimed that the Home Office sometimes over-rule their recommendations; the difficulties encountered by restricted patients from the ethnic minorities could not simply be laid at the door of the medical profession.

A question was raised about the context in which ethnic monitoring could be most useful in the provision of better treatment services. It was stated that many nurses reported anecdotally that Afro-Caribbean patients were more assaultive and difficult to manage than their white counterparts, leading to particular problems for hospitals, and especially secure units, dealing with some inner city populations. Could research in this area be effective if it only set out to show these nurses that their judgment was based on racist preconceptions? Creating the conditions in which research could foster good practice involved encouraging a sympathetic professional atmosphere in which the claims and perceptions of nurses were taken seriously and researched in an open-minded way. In a situation where nurses have to deal quickly with very difficult patients, both white and black, and where emotions can consequently run high, the task of separating out the influence of racist attitudes was necessarily complicated. It could only occur where practitioners felt that the research exercise was concerned with promoting patient care rather than with exposing how wrong they had been. Profound cultural issues needed to be addressed here which did not fall across the black/white divide. There may be a disproportionate number of black patients in inner city secure units, but the nursing and medical staff were themselves a very diverse ethnic mix.

Tackling racist attitudes

The question was raised of the significance of training in modifying racist attitudes among practitioners. Some argued against the approach of including a 'racial awareness' component in training courses, preferring that multi-cultural practices be built in to all aspects of training. Others warned against focusing feelings and perceptions, preferring to focus on structures and procedures. It was suggested that far-reaching changes outside psychiatry and the criminal justice system would ultimately have to occur in the social images of ethnic groups, as presented in advertisements and literature for instance, before wrong assumptions about differences were finally resolved.

The use of statistics to demonstrate biases was suggested as one way of undermining racist attitudes. Magistrates could be given detailed figures broken down into numbers remanded into custody, and sentenced. Dr Crowe commented that he had presented such statistics to magistrates who responded by denying that the practices occurred in their court. He called for more multi-cultural benches. Mr Francis argued that having more black magistrates and psychiatrists was not the solution, because black professionals had absorbed the dominant ways of thinking. The problems were cultural rather than about membership of particular ethnic groups.

For magistrates, a primary task was identified of raising the level of awareness that there was a subject to be understood. The ways in which society endemically predisposes a disadvantage towards blacks was something that could be demonstrated, and which could then be taken into account. A series of practical issues needed to be tackled. Why were blacks reluctant to use probation hostels, with the result that they ended up in custody? What was the relevance of cannabis abuse in the psychoses of some young black schizophrenics?

Increased representation of ethnic minorities in the criminal justice professions may be desirable, but it was pointed out that equality of opportunity was easier to achieve in the field of employment than in service delivery.

Notes

1. We would like to express our gratitude to Sashi Sashidharan, Marcia Rice and Karen Fergus whose advice, encouragement and patience was invaluable during the preparation of this paper. Needless to say, we accept full ownership of any errors.
2. Unless otherwise specified, the term 'black' is used in this paper to signify Caribbean-born, Asians, African people and British people of Caribbean extraction.
3. Property offences were defined in this instance as including theft, handling, forgery and criminal damage. Personal offences include assault, actual bodily harm, attempted robbery, threatening behaviour, indecent exposure, indecent assault and rape. Other offences included breach of the peace, drugs, obstructions, driving offences and breach of probation.

9

A view from the probation service

G. W. SMITH

Writing this paper on the mentally disordered offender, I became increasingly aware of both the importance and priority of the subject, together with the paucity of information which the probation service possessed and the neglect experienced; a disastrous combination. I became aware in my probation area of how some staff possessed both the knowledge base and the skills to make an important contribution to this area of work and yet the organization itself had not really thought through the consequences of, or the need for, a coherent system of management to deal with the problem. I learned of good local teamworking relationships which now exist between psychiatry, probation and the courts and which exist because of the inspiration of working operational staff. But I wondered why management had so rarely taken an initiative in this area when for some time I have been most certainly aware, as a chief probation officer, of the major problems that the mentally disordered offender presents to the criminal justice system.

Working in Central London one cannot help but notice an increase in mad 'Bedlam type' behaviour in the streets; to note from the service incident book that disturbed mentally ill offenders are increasingly common in our offices; to reflect on the fact that in our courts, sentencers constantly seek our help with the mentally ill defendant. Yet resources are generally lacking with the result that such defendants are more likely to end up in custody certainly at the remand stage. This was brought home to me during an experiment the Inner London Probation Service conducted in Wormwood Scrubs which looked at reducing the use of remands in custody. If you were a woman, a black defendant, or mentally disordered, you were in trouble in terms of the facilities that could be organized on your behalf to persuade a court to give you bail. If you were all three you were a walking disaster area.

Why has the probation service generally speaking neglected its responsibilities with the mentally disordered offender? I think there are two major reasons. The first is that the *Mental Health Act* 1983 placed on the social services responsibility for dealing with the mentally ill. Almost it seems, with a sigh of relief, the probation service withdrew much of its interest and commitment. This led to the second reason which I believe gathered its momentum from the liberal '60s that the offender who was 'bad' should be separated from the offender who was mentally ill. The same sort of splitting occurred unhelpfully with the *Children and Young Persons Act* 1969 when to avoid the stigma of criminalization, juveniles were to be treated as children not as offenders. It was far too simple a classification and was unhelpful to practitioners who often needed to focus on the offending behaviour to achieve effective results rather than the age of the juvenile.

This separation, as in the case of the mentally disordered offender, between the 'bad' and the 'mad' couldn't work because offenders could quite easily possess both characteristics, and indeed Bowden considers that the mentally abnormal offender has more in common with other offenders than with mentally ill patients (Bowden, 1983). But the split allowed the probation service to be both pushed and to itself withdraw from the work, which I believe only made things worse. One thing we do know about the criminal justice system is that it is in crisis partly because none of the so-called partners to the system; the police, the Crown Prosecution Service, the courts, the probation service, the Prison Department, seem rarely prepared or able to work together. Far too often they set up their own individual defences and value system which work one against the other. The recent Green Paper *Punishment, Custody and the Community* (Home Office, 1988*b*) crucially emphasized partnership as the only way we can all move forward.

The same lack of partnership is evident for the mentally disordered offender. The current trend in the health service towards community care and the closing of mental hospitals has occurred against an environment in which the receiving communities possess neither the resources, the willingness nor the understanding to receive them. The further consequences of this disharmony upon other agencies, such as those in the criminal justice system, with the increase in the number of mentally disordered people appearing before courts and, if current practice continues, in custody, have not been appreciated until recently.

The tendency to withdraw from the subject of mentally disordered offenders has also allowed the probation service to claim too often that it now lacks the expertise to deal with the problem. I have been concerned how often staff express an unwillingness to deal with the mentally disordered. I often hear the claim that it is someone else's responsibility. There is the suggestion that they are too dangerous and we don't have the resources to deal with them. Hostels are reluctant to accept the mentally ill as residents and there is an absence of specialist hostels dealing with this problem that probation officers can refer to. Such lack of facilities reinforces the reluctance of staff to deal with the mentally disordered. A recent study of London bail hostels states that most wardens feel they 'lack the resources to deal with the mentally disturbed offender' (Home Office, 1979).

However, the hostels that will take the mentally disordered too often seem to put their needs before that of the resident/patient. Admission procedures can take an agonizingly long time, and they also tend not to welcome short stays and by short I mean less that one year. Often it is crucial for treatment to move a person on through a residential setting to independent living. The hostel that is reluctant to let a patient go to the next stage is not uncommon.

I am also concerned about the disadvantages that patients experience who have been in receipt of sickness benefit for 28 weeks. Whilst they will get the invalidity benefit automatically which gives them more than income supplement, it disqualifies them for a community care grant. This means they are deprived of one of the few discretionary payments left in the system, money which could be available to provide furniture, clothes etc, to set them up with some chance of success after a long stay in an institution.

Over the past 18 months, one of the few positive features has been the way the probation service has increased its activity in the pre-court situation. It has done this to reduce both the number of people appearing in court and the use of remands in custody. This has become possible with the introduction of the Crown Prosecution Service. Their arrival on the criminal justice scene has provided us with the opportunity to divert offenders out of the system altogether, thus reducing overall the net widening effect which, if unchecked, leads to defendants rising too rapidly and unfairly up the sentencing tariff ladder. The Crown Prosecution Service can discontinue a case if they judge it to be in the public interest and one of the criteria they can use is that of mental illness. They are therefore a crucial new ingredient in the concerted attempt we can all make in keeping a significant percentage of mentally disordered offenders out of the criminal justice system.

The Crown Prosecution Service also make the recommendation to courts as to whether a defendant should receive bail or not. More use of bailing people to the community rather than custody would have a significant effect on our prison overcrowding crisis. Research also shows that a defendant if convicted is more likely to receive a custodial sentence if he has already been held on remand in custody. Anything that can break this vicious cycle is therefore to be welcomed. If the probation officer can offer services at this stage for the mentally disordered defendant such as hostel or other community care, they are likely to be able to make a very positive impact on the situation.

Interestingly, there appears to be a significant difference between the numbers of mentally disordered in custody at the remand as opposed to the post-sentence stages. Whilst the evidence appears to suggest that the incidence of mental disorder at the post-sentence stage is about average for the normal population, Taylor and Gunn's study at Brixton showed a significantly higher prevalence of disorder within the remand population (Taylor & Gunn, 1984a;b). Additionally, Taylor in her study of London life sentence offenders showed a high rate of psychiatric disorder within this group whether the lifers were in prison or in the community (Taylor, 1986). Two-thirds of her sample in this study had a psychiatric diagnosis, 10% had schizophrenia and a slightly higher proportion a depressive illness. Of her sample, nearly one-third of those released had to be recalled to prison because of 'adjustment problems' rather than re-offending.

It is probably worth pausing at this point to reflect on the problems facing the mentally disordered offender in the criminal justice system. The first obvious one is that the prison service is not equipped or able to deal with the mentally ill. Pobation officers in prisons are frequently asked to deal with inmates whose behaviour is bizarre and not infrequently dangerous either to themselves or others. Medication and treatment is either non-existent or inappropriate and the mentally ill have to share cells with others not themselves ill, which provides mutual distress and the possibility of unfair advantage being taken.

There is a tendency, understandably I suppose, for staff and other inmates to become exasperated with the mentally disordered which can add to their distress and difficulties. This also spills into the criminal justice system outside. It is often difficult to get a solicitor to take on such cases where the offender is obviously behaving in a bizarre way.

The Prison Medical Service, with its overcrowding problem, finds it difficult to provide adequate psychiatric reports on many of these offenders and the frustration and sense of inadequacy is compounded when the defendant arrives at a court which knows something needs to be done but does not know what or how to go about it.

The mentally disordered individual outside the institution generally has more problems with accommodation, with coping, with employment, than the remainder of the community. There is an absence of support for them with their problems and they can too easily slip into crime to resolve them.

So what can the probation service do? The first focus for their activity should be through the extension and creation of cautioning, diversion, and bail information schemes keeping the mentally disordered offender out of the courts and custody altogether. This requires partnership with the psychiatric service as well as police, Crown Prosecution Service and the courts, something which I have already commented is most conspicuous so far by its absence. So a direct involvement in more cautioning and diversion by psychiatric services would appear to be a sensible investment. I have already mentioned involvement with the Crown Prosecution Service at the stage at which they can discontinue cases if they feel it is not in the public interest.

Another area is in the provision of bail information schemes which are now being established by probation services throughout the country. They have a tremendous potential for being helpful to the mentally disordered. A common precipitant of custody is the lack of a fixed address or accommodation. As we know this is a particular problem for many mentally disordered offenders, we also know that this is one of the major reasons why they end up in custody even though their offence in itself might not warrant it. The mentally disordered often lack other support systems and suffer from the lack of understanding and even fear that bizarre behaviour can create in others who are psychiatrically normal; police often perceive the mentally disordered as more dangerous. The element of self-harm which may exist also can cause courts to place in custody on the basis that it is for the offender's own good even though the overall effect is likely to be far worse for everyone.

The sentencer's problem in such matters is further reinforced by the obvious and real inability of police, probation services, and social services to provide adequate compensatory facilities for the mentally disordered offender. Until this is rectified, the situation is likely to remain very difficult.

The Head of the Greater London bail information scheme says that concern for the mentally ill has been mentioned at every meeting she has established with police, Crown Prosecution Service, magistrates, court clerks and solicitors. 'Can the probation service do anything to help?' – 'We have to remand in custody because there is nowhere else'. These are constant comments. As part of the bail information process, probation officers will be monitoring the extent of the psychiatric and medical problems which they experience. It should give us some idea of the extent of the problems with which we are faced.

I believe that the Home Office who are paying for the 'care' of NHS patients needs to actively and firmly divert back to the medical system those who should receive treatment and support within the community. The appropriate implementation of the Griffiths Report with funding for non-criminal justice accommodation needs to be pursued (Griffiths, 1988). The collaboration this requires is not helped by the fact that health authority boundaries do not coincide with court boundaries. One of my dreams is that criminal justice, health and education could all work to the same administrative boundaries. Is it a far-fetched dream? It would certainly not be particularly difficult to achieve. We so often tinker meaninglessly with local authority boundaries, and it would certainly aid matters.

Another scheme, and one of the most encouraging in dealing with the problem, is a partnership being operated between local psychiatric services and the probation service at the three central London courts of Bow Street, Marlborough Street and Horseferry Road. By nature of their location, these courts have a high number of seriously ill defendants cluttering up court time although, by and large, they are not serious offenders.

Under this scheme, the duty probation officer identifies appropriate cases who are then seen by a duty psychiatrist. The psychiatrist will then prepare a report for the court and also frequently will be able to offer either in-patient or out-patient treatment. One important spin-off is how the presence of the psychiatrist gives confidence to probation service and sentencer to take risks because they perceive there is appropriate medical 'back-up' on call. Additionally, the consultant psychiatrists offer an advisory service to the probation staff in respect of those of their cases who are mentally ill. I observed one such consultation in progress. What impressed me was the willingness of probation officers to work with the mentally disordered offender, and the confidence the consultant gave them both in the appropriateness of what they were doing and the results they could achieve. Such a partnership presumes that the existence of such schemes would lead to hostels being more willing to take the mentally disordered offender if they could be assured that they were 'safe' and that speedy 'back-up' was guaranteed if anything went wrong. They also believe that, if it was possible for a psychiatrist to be available to court, a bail hostel would be willing to accept referrals who were mentally ill if initial psychiatric assessment was guaranteed within 24 hours, and first stay at the hostel limited to 72 or 96 hours. I agree with them.

For the probation service, therefore, working with the mentally disordered offender can only succeed if there is this meaningful liaison between itself and psychiatry. In the Netherlands, most probation teams have the regular support of their own consultant psychiatrist. We need more such formal arrangements in the United Kingdom. An increase in the number of probation officers working in secure units would also be desirable. The information and skill they can gather would be important for the service. The North East London probation project with two probation officers and two psychiatrists offering out-patient groups for paedophiles is another good example of what can be achieved, and there is considerable scope here for further development. I am certainly interested in the possibility of a specialized bail hostel for the mentally disordered which would be jointly staffed by probation and medical staff. The Denis Hill Unit have ideas about such a development.

There is obviously a tremendous need to be met, and where the probation service has made a deliberate attempt to work with the problem, the 'take-up' by the court has been considerable. A recent example is the study by the community resources team at Borough High Street (Hale, 1989). They were testing the hypothesis that homeless offenders appearing at Horseferry Road Court could be dealt with by probation rather than custody if the social inquiry report made the appropriate recommendation. Of the sample of offenders 41% were mentally disordered, but in 73% of the cases a probation order was made. What was a little worrying was whether the probation order was the right disposal for this group and whether it added to the risk of criminalization for defendants who were essentially mentally ill. But what was fascinating about the study, and against the perceived wisdom, was that a chaotic, homeless, alcoholic, mentally disordered group could keep appointments and respond to supervision.

I would also wish to see improved contact between psychiatry and probation services where there is a condition in the order for treatment. This has been allowed to drift, and far too often I see 'separate track' working of the order. So often patients break down because they stop taking their medication and yet nothing happens. The side-effects of drugs may well be the loss of initiative and spontaneity. The patients' quality of life appears poor. I regret that the essential degree of professional closeness necessary to deal with this problem has not been fully grasped by either of our services.

Angus Cameron, who has been a great help to me in the working of this paper and who is a probation officer working in the Denis Hill Unit, has drawn together criteria for establishing when work with the mentally disordered offender should be the responsibility of the probation service. It goes as follows and certainly I would commend it.

The probation service should accept responsibility:

(i)   if in the community – where the mentally disordered offender has a significant history of offending or significant contact with the probation service;
(ii) if in-patient – where the probation service has had significant knowledge/contact prior to admission;
(iii) where patient has significant criminal history;
(iv) for patients subject to a restriction order under s.41 or s.49 of *Mental Health Act* 1983;
(v)   for patients transferred from prison to psychiatric hospitals under s.47 of Mental Health Act 1983;
(vii) for patients who have been remanded from court or remand prison to hospital and are still subject to court process.

In conclusion there appears to be a number of issues which the probation service should concern itself with to deal effectively with the mentally disordered offender:

(i)   Close formal working relationships with psychiatrists during pre-court cautioning. Diversion and bail information schemes.
(ii) A similar relationship and formal arrangement to provide jointly a social inquiry report and information service to defendants who are mentally ill appearing in court.
(iii) The provision of specialized bail facilities for the remand population plus speedily available 'back-up' services for treatment and help.
(iv) Formal consultancy service by psychiatrists, services for probation teams working in high risk areas.
(v)   More transfers between prisons and ordinary psychiatric hospitals.

(vi) More joint funding between Home Office and health departments in respect of the mentally disordered offenders.
(vii) More direct involvement by the probation service in regional secure units.

10

A view from the prison medical service

R. J. WOOL

In any society, problems abound whose histories contain all the hallmarks of a chronic condition; chronic because underlying causes were not searched out or, if they were, there was a failure adequately to tackle them. That failure may have stemmed from a view that the problem was small enough to live with, could be isolated, or was simply too difficult to contemplate. In varying degrees, it has been the lot of the mentally disturbed to suffer in this way.

Attitudes may be improving. Certainly there is no lack of attention drawn to the question of how and where to deliver proper levels of care. Increasingly, government policy points to this being in the community rather than in large Victorian psychiatric hospitals. The policy of care in the community has philosophical implications for society's response to mentally disordered people who commit offences. Perhaps more particularly, it may have – or indeed be having – important practical implications for the prison service. Medical journals are no strangers to articles purporting to show a causal link between the implementation of the care in the community policy and the number of mentally disordered offenders in prison.

The absence of hard proof of such a link does nothing to diminish the proper anxiety about the number of mentally disturbed people the courts sent to prison, and the provision which the prison service has thus far been able to provide. There will be few who quarrel with either strand of the government's policy, which first looks to the diversion of such people from the criminal justice system (Home Office, 1990a); and, where custody is deemed to be in the public interest, expects an appropriate level of support to be provided for them from within the prison system. There is much scope for the development of responses to both.

Many openings short of custody exist for dealing with mentally disordered offenders. The police may apply a caution and may themselves – perhaps in conjunction with the social services – arrange admission to hospital or help in the community. The courts have available a wide range of non-custodial disposals. They can remand on bail with a condition of residence at a psychiatric hospital or bail hostel. They can remand direct to hospital for psychiatric reports. In cases of mental illness or severe mental impairment, the Crown Court may remand to hospital for treatment. And where a prisoner on remand is diagnosed as suffering from such a form of mental disorder, and is in need of urgent treatment, the Home Secretary can direct his immediate transfer to hospital. There is, too, the possibility of making a probation order with a requirement of psychiatric treatment, either as a resident or as a non-resident.

Diversion requires not only commitment on the part of those with the power to arrange it, but their clear understanding of these powers and the facilities available. Means need to be found of providing the courts with swifter initial diagnoses. There is a need, too, for more facilities in the community covering a comprehensive range; from more places in regional secure units to facilities where the disturbed or bewildered can take refuge. The inter-departmental working group of Home Office and Department of Health officials considered some of these issues in its 1987 report (Home Office, 1987b). The Departments have prepared a wide-ranging circular aimed at encouraging better co-operation between the courts, police, probation services and other agencies responsible for dealing with mentally disturbed offenders (Home Office, 1990a). There are a number of initiatives directed at reducing numbers in custody. A consultative paper issued in February 1989 paved the way for further consideration of the contribution which hostels could make (Home Office, 1989b).

Proof of the need for such focused activity is easy to come by. A visit to any busy local prison immediately provides evidence of numbers of mentally disturbed defendants ill-matched by the resources available to attend them. There are hard statistics too. The number of psychiatric reports requested from prison medical officers by the courts has steadily fallen over the years. Figures 10.1 and 10.2 show that, in 1979, 9384 such reports were prepared. In 1988/89, the numbers stood at 6384 (both figures include a few hundred offered voluntarily by prison medical officers even though the reports had not been requested). It is also of interest that some reports prepared by prison medical officers are in respect of defendants' bail applications. The preparation of reports

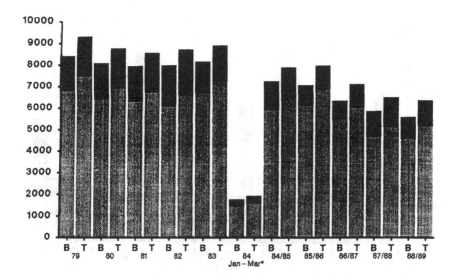

Fig. 10.1. Psychiatric reports by medical officers. 'B' = Number of psychiatric reports by medical officers on persons remanded in custody. 'T' = Total number of psychiatric medical reports to Court. * Change from calendar to financial years; ▨, 21 and over; ■, under 21.

remains a major task at Brixton Prison, where the reduction has been much less marked, with the prison preparing over 35% (2200) of the national total of reports in 1988/89.

Problems exist not only in obtaining beds for certain groups of offender – in particular those likely to require long-term secure accommodation but who do not merit allocation to a special hospital. Some hospital transfers take too long to arrange. It may take several weeks before a consultant psychiatrist is able to visit a prison to see and prepare a report on a patient. Returns obtained from prison medical officers over a three month period in 1989 point to 25% of assessment visits taking between two and four weeks to achieve, and 8% longer than that. I cannot avoid a sense of concern that the Mental Health Act Code of Practice regards it as essential for a nurse to accompany the doctor where admission to hospital is likely to be recommended (Department of Health, 1990). The value of the underlying purpose is evident enough. But will some delays become more protracted?

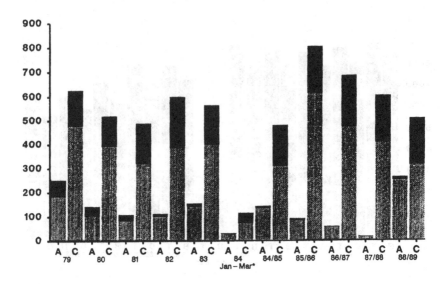

Fig. 10.2. Psychiatric reports by medical officers. 'A' = Number of psychiatric reports by medical officers on persons remanded on bail. 'C' = Number of reports voluntarily submitted by medical officers. * Change from calendar to financial years; ▨, 21 and over; ■, under 21.

This is not to overlook weaknesses closer to home. Forthcoming revised instructions to governors and medical officers will emphasize the importance of action being taken as early as possible to initiate the various procedures designed in appropriate cases to secure a patient's removal to hospital. This may entail some flexibility in prison routines when an early visit by a consultant psychiatrist cannot otherwise be accommodated.

The annual number of offenders removed to hospital by the courts following the reports by prison medical officers has remained roughly the same over the ten-year period. Figure 10.3 shows that it stood at 869 in 1979, reached a peak of 907 in 1983 and in 1988/89 fell to 803 (but was 880 in 1987/88).

Also of note is the trend in probation orders with a requirement of psychiatric treatment. In 1979, 1430 persons commenced such supervision. There was a peak of 1700 in 1980. In 1988 the figure was 980 – a 40% reduction from the 1980 peak. Small wonder that people working in prison argue from direct experience that the minor offender who requires

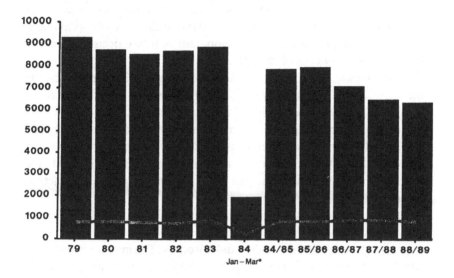

Fig. 10.3. Court orders arising from prison medical officers' reports. *Change from calendar to financial years; ■ number of medical officers' reports; ▓, number of court orders.

neither custody nor removal to hospital features increasingly amongst the inmate population.

Coid, in a retrospective survey of mentally abnormal men remanded to Winchester Prison for psychiatric reports over the years 1979–83, found that one in five were rejected for treatment by the NHS consultant psychiatrist responsible for their care (Coid, 1988a). He states that 'Those with mental handicaps, organic brain damage, or a chronic psychotic illness rendering them unable to cope independently in the community were the most likely to be rejected. They posed the least threat to the community in terms of their criminal behaviour yet were more likely to be sentenced to imprisonment.'

Conversely, the annual number of transfers from prison to hospital under the provisions of the *Mental Health Act* 1983 made on the direction of the Secretary of State has doubled to 200 over the last ten years which I believe provides further evidence of the commitment of the Prison Medical Service. Over recent years the number of the cases accepted annually by the special hospitals has been in the order of 55, which, together with notable refusals, caused concern that the admission procedures failed in their primary tasks. The recent establishment of the Special Hospitals Service Authority, and initial contacts with its management, hold the promise of the development of future decisions more in keeping with the needs of the patient.

While the social services, the police and the courts have major roles in the diversion of mentally disturbed offenders, the reality has to be accepted that many are received into prison custody. Like it or not, all those working within the prison environment must do the best they can for them. I see no profound philosophical or intellectual problems in the strategy to meet that acceptance. Possible solutions are essentially based on pragmatic considerations, just as impediments are of a practical nature.

Existing specialist establishments, of which Grendon is of course the prime example, have a major part to play. This contribution is not only in respect of the help afforded individual prisoners. The manner and style of such help present an example to service managers and other staff of an alternative means of maintaining security and control over a population of serious offenders with the maximum of involvement and a minimum of force and coercion. In discussing the treatment of mentally disturbed offenders in the prison context, I believe it to be unnecessary and potentially unhelpful to indulge in a close examination of the *Mental Health Act* 1983 or other definitions. If the given position is that a person in prison custody who is detainable within the meaning of the Mental Health Act is, eventually, so detained, energies can be concentrated on those whose length of stay within prison is a reflection of the courts' sentence.

Many people are in custody because of behavioural problems neither they nor agencies in the community have confronted. Such problems may present in one or more of a range of anti-social acts including those of violence and addiction. A recent study, commissioned by the Prison Department, of the three adult male therapy wings at Grendon psychiatric prison found that the patients were typically serving long sentences for crimes of sex or violence with a significant proportion previously on Rule 43 (Genders & Player, 1989). This was markedly different from the characteristics prevailing during Professor Gunn's study in the 1970s when the patients were at the lighter end of the market, with a much higher proportion of what are described as recidivist property offenders (Gunn *et al.*, 1978). Only 32% of the 1971–72 receptions were serving sentences for offences of violence against the person, including sexual offences and robbery. This contrasts with 81% of the 1987–88 receptions. Virtually all of the recent receptions were serving sentences of more than three years. The study contains helpful pointers to areas and ways in which planning and provision might be further developed. It exposes, too, the need for improved arrangements for the patient's release back into the community, and his continuing support there. I hope the study, which is being carefully considered by the Advisory Committee on the therapeutic regime at Grendon, will also nail the myth that time at Grendon is a soft option. It is apparent now more than previously that Grendon, an excellent example of a multi-disciplinary environment, scoring both in the level of help given disturbed individuals and the part it plays in humanely containing some very difficult offenders, is both challenging in the personal demands it makes of the patients and able to flex its muscles as a measure of last resort.

In reviewing related policies, the Prisons' Board endorsed the view that specialized establishments have a vital place in its overall strategy but are not the sole model for a continued response by the service to mentally disturbed prisoners, whatever the crime which brought them to notice. Essential to the development of policy was an objective assessment of the size and nature of the problem, the facilities in place and what might be needed to meet the assumed shortfall. For that purpose Professor Gunn was commissioned to produce a psychiatric profile of the sentenced population. His three year study has recently been published (Gunn *et al.*, 1991).

Consideration of the problems faced by the service in coping with the needs of such offenders clearly indicated that policy could not stand still. The Board endorsed the principles that inmates' state of mental health would be a prime factor in routine, in-service allocation decisions; and that in each prison service region there would be selected a small number of establishments which progressively would be geared towards managing that sector of the inmate population. The modest prison facilities available for coping with mentally disturbed inmates gives an odd ring to the statement required by a select committee that there is no intention of developing facilities which would duplicate those in psychiatric hospitals (UK Government, 1987). The standards to which I hope we shall be working in these establishments are simply expressed as being on a par with out-patient treatment. But that, too, is misleading. I see the relatively small additional numbers of psychiatrically trained staff, when we can get them, adopting a consultancy or supporting role for the general run of prison staff in regular contact with the inmate.

It will thus be the generality of staff who will increasingly develop the attitudes and skills necessary to care for disturbed inmates, fortified through the learning and experience of highly trained specialists, only a few of whom would be located in the prison hospital. In the order of 40% of prison medical officers have a psychiatric qualification. The desperate need is for more hospital officers and nurses with psychiatric qualifications and experience. Recruitment is well short of target, and calls for a hard look both at the level of effort and skill the department applies to the task and whether the policy of unification of the hospital and nursing grades creates a barrier.

The prison service has thus set for itself not so much a new direction but a multiple approach; enhancing the scope of existing specialist facilities, with particular reference to Grendon, while simultaneously developing the service's capability to care for mentally disordered offenders, at a lower level of intensity, in selected establishments in each region. We shall need the support of a wide range of practitioners and policy makers in progressing towards these objectives. In particular, our task will be all the harder if the flow of mentally disturbed people sent to prison – by no means all of whom are there in the public interest – continues unabated.

What need – or chance – of a second Grendon? I would foresee no shortage of clients. The recent study points to a waiting list approximating to the current level of occupancy. Its value for patients is clear and for the service in general. But it is undoubtedly costly in resources. In concluding that there was not then a sufficiently strong case for establishing a second psychiatric prison, the Butler Committee pointed to the risk of the demands that would be made on scarce resources being prejudicial to treatment in other prisons (Home Office/DHSS, 1975). That would remain my very real concern. But the next step is to consider the implications of Professor Gunn's research.

11

A view from the courts: diversion and discontinuance

P. JOSEPH

Introduction

In 1967 a study was carried out examining women remanded for medical reports to Holloway Prison (Dell & Gibbens, 1971). Less than 9% received a hospital order and not more than another 10% were sentenced to imprisonment or borstal training. Thus 80% of the women sent to prison for medical examination were released into the community after the remand period. The most likely reason was that the time spent on remand in custody had exceeded the likely punishment for the offence. Gibbens *et al.* (1977) went on to describe the medical remand procedure in some detail and to compare the court practices in London and Wessex. He found that, in London, magistrates remanded more defendants for medical reports and a disproportionate number of those were remanded in custody. However, smaller numbers of the London defendants received a hospital order or a probation order with a condition of treatment compared with those in Wessex. One conclusion drawn from this study was that the busier the court the more likely a remand in custody for medical reports. Bowden (1978) studied a sample of men remanded into custody for medical reports during a three month period in 1975. He described a recidivist population with previous offences for theft, drunkenness, vagrancy and violence, with frequent short periods of imprisonment. He noted they had similar characteristics to habitual drunken offenders and vagrants. A medical recommendation was associated with presence of mental illness and previous admissions to psychiatric hospital, and an absence of alcohol abuse or an extensive criminal record. His assertion that hospitals would only accept the better risk cases is supported by Binns *et al.* (1969) who compared mentally disordered offenders who were remanded to hospital under s.54 of the *Mental Health (Scotland) Act* 1960 with those medically remanded in custody.

Has the situation changed since those studies were carried out? The answer depends on which prison is looked at. For example, at Holloway Prison the picture has changed dramatically since Dell and Gibbens' study carried out in 1967. Over the three years 1986–1989 approximately 20–25% of medical remands have received a hospital placement. For the period April 1988 to March 1989 of 516 medical assessments, there was 136 placements in hospital (N. Hindson, personal communication), a rate of 26% which is far in excess of the figure of 9% found by Dell and Gibbens. One reason for this may be the increasing willingness by the medical staff at Holloway Prison to provide a voluntary report, rather than only providing reports requested by the court. In contrast, at Brixton Prison for the period April 1988 to March 1989 there were 2217 psychiatric reports submitted by medical officers, 35% of the total for England and Wales, of which 211 resulted in hospital placement, a rate of 9.5%, which is virtually unchanged from a decade ago (Home Office, 1989a).

It is clear that the vast majority of defendants who are remanded into custody for medical reports do not subsequently go to hospital. What is the function of such a remand? Scott (1967) suggested that the courts' intentions might be punitive, but this probably only applied to a minority of cases. It is more likely that the remand prison serves a number of different functions. Faulk and Trafford (1975) suggested it functioned as a simple bail hostel for those defendants who found themselves with no fixed address, as a secure bail hostel for those who had already broken bail, as an acute alcoholic admission unit for those who required medical supervision while drying out from severe alcohol abuse, and as an acute psychiatric ward for those with severe mental disturbance. In addition to those functions, custody represents a convenient storage facility to allow a psychiatric assessment to take place.

Why is the option of bail not used more widely? The *Bail Act* 1976 recognizes the right of a defendant to be granted bail unless one of a number of objections apply. For the homeless mentally ill petty offender, bail is usually refused on two grounds: lack of community ties and for the protection of the defendant. The first objection might be overcome if there were more bail hostels, but the recent Green Paper 'Private Sector Involvement in the Remand System' (Home Office, 1988a) recognizes that bail hostels may refuse a place to a defendant who is mentally disordered or who has an extensive psychiatric history. The second objection to bail may even apply to those mentally disordered offenders who have been charged with a non-imprisonable offence; this is one of the few exceptions to the rule that the offence must be imprisonable in order to remand into custody.

Psychiatric assessment service

It is apparent that a combination of factors is resulting in an excessive number of defendants being remanded in custody for medical reports. Not only is this wasteful of court and prison resources, but more importantly it is a serious infringement of personal liberty, especially when some of those remanded into custody have been charged with non-imprisonable offences. The current procedure of psychiatric assessment at prison is grossly inefficient. There is often insufficient time to assess the defendant before the next appearance in court and indeed, great concern has been expressed at the number of prisoners locked out of the prisons and kept in police custody. The figure was 800 in November 1988. This meant that the defendant was often not back at the prison before his next appearance in court, thus leading to a merry-go-round of court appearances, followed by a further remand in custody. When the psychiatrist was able to catch up with the prisoner there was often limited time available for assessment and very little information about the nature of the charge, the defendant's previous convictions, etc. It is difficult to envisage how an assessment of dangerousness and treatability can be made with any confidence on the basis of one prison visit.

Bearing these problems in mind, a psychiatric assessment service has now been in operation at two inner London magistrates' courts since February 1989. The two courts in question, Bow Street and Marlborough Street, are extremely busy, proceeding with 20 000 persons in 1987. Because of the areas they serve, many homeless mentally ill and petty offenders appear before magistrates who are often at a loss to know how to deal with them. A psychiatric on-call service is available during two sessions per week and referrals are accepted from the magistrates, probation officers, duty solicitor, or sometimes the police officers in the gaolers' area. The assessment of the defendant is made in the gaolers' area at the court, usually in the probation officer's or duty solicitor's room, or occasionally in the cell itself; interviews are very rarely conducted through the cell window. Following psychiatric assessment, if admission to hospital is indicated an approved social worker and second doctor are readily available to attend. Following completion of the assessment and the securing of a hospital bed, the psychiatrist provides a verbal report to the court which allows for further questioning by the magistrates if required.

The advantages of this scheme are as follows:

(a) There is a great deal more information available to the psychiatrist because he has access to the Crown Prosecution Service file which gives details of the charge, witness statements and previous convictions of the defendant.
(b) The duty probation officer is available to provide background information, if available, and to discuss options, for example bail hostels.
(c) The duty solicitor is available to discuss issues regarding entering a plea, and of course the defendant is always available, having not been diverted to a different prison for example.
(d) The most important advantage is the opportunity for a discussion to take place between the psychiatrist, magistrate and Crown Prosecution Service regarding the suitability of discontinuing the case, which is fundamental to the success or otherwise of this scheme.

Results

Demographic characteristics of 80 consecutive patients referred to the psychiatrist are described in Table 11.1. The population is predominantly male and unattached both in terms of accommodation and stable relationships. Many have migrated to London from other parts of Great Britain. The offences with which they are charged tend to be minor (Table 11.2). Fourteen cases had been charged with a non-imprisonable public order offence. Only one case, robbery, was being committed to the Crown Court. Twenty-one per cent had no previous convictions. The defendants fell into two groups, those who are assessed pre-trial (75%), usually within one week of arrest, and the remainder who had been remanded into custody for medical reports, but no report was available.

The primary diagnoses are shown in Table 11.3. Of the sample, 77% had previously been psychiatric in-patients, the majority detained under civil or criminal provisions of the *Mental Health Act* 1983. Only 5% had no mental disorder, a figure which reflects the appropriateness of the referrals.

The medical recommendations are shown in Table 11.4. In all cases where a hospital disposal was recommended and a bed was available, the court complied. For those defendants admitted to hospital either informally or under a civil section of the *Mental Health Act* 1983, $n = 24$

Table 11.1. *Demographic characteristics of 80 consecutive defendants (numbers and percentages)*

	N	%		N	%
Sex			*Place of birth*		
Male	65	81	London	18	23
Female	15	19	Scotland	4	5
			North England	13	16
Age			Rest of England and Wales	19	24
20–30	40	50	Ireland	4	5
31–40	23	28	Caribbean	7	9
41+	17	22	Africa	5	6
			Other	10	12
Marital status					
Single	62	77	*Accommodation*		
Married	3	4	Streets	39	49
Separated/divorced	15	29	Hostel	12	15
			Squat	6	8
Ethnic origin			Settled	23	28
Caucasian	52	65			
Afro-Caribbean	19	24			
Asian	6	7			
Mixed race	3	4			

Table 11.2. *Offences* with which 80 consecutive defendants were charged (numbers and percentages)*

	N	%
Public order	28	35
Theft	13	16
Non-payment of meal	7	9
Assault	12	15
Criminal damage	11	14
Offensive weapon	8	10
Indecent exposure	5	6
Breach of bail	5	6
Annoying phone calls	3	4
Other	4	5

* Some defendants were charged with more than one offence.

Table 11.3. *Primary diagnosis of the sample (numbers and percentages)*

	N	%
Schizophrenia	38	47
Affective psychosis	9	11
Drug induced psychosis	5	6
Alcohol dependence	5	6
Dementia	1	1
Neurotic disorder	4	5
Personality disorder	8	10
Uncertain	6	7
No mental disorder	4	5

Table 11.4. *Medical recommendations for the sample (numbers and percentages)*

	N	%
None	29	36
Psychiatric out-patient attendance	21	26
Probation and out-patient treatment	2	2
Informal admission to hospital	5	6
Bail to hospital	4	5
Section 2 *Mental Health Act* 1983 admission to hospital	11	15
Section 3 *Mental Health Act* 1983 admission to hospital	1	1
Section 35 *Mental Health Act* 1983 admission to hospital	6	8
Section 37 *Mental Health Act* 1983 admission to hospital	1	1

(30%), the case was discontinued by the Crown Prosecution Service. A further four (5%) cases were discontinued without a recommendation for hospital admission, giving a total discontinuance rate of 35%. Forty-one (51%) defendants were released into the community following psychiatric assessment leaving only 15 (19%) who were returned to custody, mainly due to administrative difficulties in arranging immediate hospital admission.

Case illustration

Christine, aged 23 years, arrived in London from the north of England in December 1988, and was living rough and not claiming benefit, preferring to live on the streets than in hostels. Over the next four months she was arrested seven times and remanded to Holloway Prison on two occasions for public order offences. Medical reports submitted on both occasions stated that she was probably of below average intelligence and did not require hospital admission. She was seen by the court psychiatrist following arrest on a charge of attempted criminal damage, having attacked a cement mixer with a wooden pole, and she was admitted to hospital from court under s.35 of the *Mental Health Act* 1983 for preparation of a psychiatric report. Whilst in hospital, florid psychotic symptoms were noted, in addition to mild mental handicap. Her previous psychiatric history revealed a two-year in-patient admission to a psychiatric hospital in the north of England following an assault on an eight year-old boy. On return to court a month later the case was discontinued and she was placed on s.3 of the *Mental Health Act* 1983 and returned to hospital where she remained six months later having shown a marked improvement. At the time of writing she is currently awaiting placement in a Richmond Fellowship Hostel.

Conclusion

There appears to be a growing commitment by the Home Office and the courts to avoid a remand in custody for medical reports whenever possible (Home Office, 1990*a*). Previous attempts, such as the use of bail clinics attached to Holloway and Brixton, were largely unsuccessful in diverting defendants from custody and the number seen were very small. Two new schemes under the direction of the probation service have recently been introduced: first, the Bail Information Service, which aims to provide the court with more information about the background and circumstances of the defendant in order to allow a more balanced view to be reached regarding the granting of bail (Stone, 1988); secondly, the Public Interest Case Assessment Scheme, which is designed to provide the Crown Prosecution Service with sufficient information to allow a decision to be made whether to discontinue the case against the defendant on the grounds that it is not in the public interest (Stone, 1989). These two schemes, coupled with a promised increase in the number of bail hostel placements will hopefully make a major impact on the numbers of defendants currently being remanded in custody.

The scheme described here fits into this pattern of diversion and discontinuance. For 35% of defendants the case against them was not proceeded with as not being in the public interest. This is allowed under s.23(3) of the *Prosecution of Offences Act* 1985 and the public interest criteria are set out in the *Code for Crown Prosecutors*. The figures are far in excess of the usual 1–2% discontinuance rate.

The impact of this scheme on hospital-based resources remains to be evaluated. Although there is likely to be an increase in the number of admissions to hospital, diversion from custody does not necessarily result in diversion to hospital as half the sample were released into the community. In addition, assessment at court should reduce the numbers of defendants requiring assessment at the prison.

The shift of the focus of psychiatric assessment in the case of mentally disordered petty offenders from the prison to court allows for the adoption of a more pragmatic and flexible response at an earlier stage of the proceedings and greater communication to take place between the criminal justice and mental health systems.

Discussion

The contributions covered a cluster of issues relating to the diversion of mentally disordered offenders from the criminal justice system and the provision of appropriate treatment at the earliest possible stage. Two implications of these requirements were followed through in the discussion; the need for agencies to relate effectively to one another and the possible need for additional resources.

Diversion and early treatment

The discussion began with a powerful plea for the early and effective treatment of mentally disordered offenders. It was argued that minor offenders, if given appropriate treatment could be prevented from proceeding with a career involving increasingly serious offences, and the responsibility for diversion into treatment and avoidance of court appearances at an early stage of the offender's criminal career could lie with the Crown Prosecution Service. Another contributor responded with scepticism about the ability of psychiatry to deliver this kind of preventative treatment (with another making the general observation that sentencers had over-inflated expectations of psychiatrists). However, efforts at preventative treatment were worthwhile, and the scheme described by

Dr Joseph was one that exemplified good practice in the rapid response of the psychiatrists.

Although one contributor recognized that modern sentencing was far more complicated than it had been in the late 1960s, with a greater range of factors having to be taken into account, and a concomitant increase in sentencing training seminars, another suggested that, in some areas, little progress had been made in the ways in which mentally disordered offenders were handled by the courts. Over 30 years ago, at the time when the late Peter Scott had been working in the field, concern had been expressed over remands in custody for psychiatric reports, with prisons seen as unsuitable places in which to make a psychiatric assessment. However, the problem remained today. It was noted that some relevant powers of mental health legislation were under-used by the courts, particularly the power to remand to hospital for a report on the defendant's mental condition (s.35 of the *Mental Health Act*, 1983). A call was made for centres to be set up within the National Health Service, which could reduce the number of remands in custody. However, Dr Joseph emphasized that diversion from prison did not necessarily imply diversion into a hospital, but could be to some provision of community care.

It was argued that remands in custody particularly disadvantaged homeless people accused of petty offences. In line with the general requirement for the provision of bail hostels and a decreasing use of remand in custody, some kind of special housing provision was required for this particular group, as was an end to prosecutions for offences of being drunk and disorderly. This would relieve the courts of the problem of dealing with these individuals, while at the same time there might be some decrease in their rate of offending. Dr Wool reminded the conference that there was still a requirement for the Prison Medical Service to initiate systems of rapid intervention within the prisons. There was greater awareness of the need to identify and treat drug abusers, and a concept of 'through care' was developing within the service.

Effective working relationships between agencies

A number of contributors commented on the ways in which different agencies should relate to one another, with the aim of achieving the diversion and rapid treatment of mentally disordered offenders. The key problem of the lack of immediate access to psychiatric services by the courts was raised. One contributor suggested that busy inner-city general psychiatrists were already under great pressure. They might see forensic issues as outside their competence, although this was not necessarily true. Forensic psychiatrists were few in number. More were needed, although even a minimal forensic presence made a difference, allowing effective liaison between general psychiatry and the forensic services, and enabling patients to be placed in forensic psychiatric facilities. Dr Joseph's scheme was unusual in so far as it was established within a post-graduate research institute. It was suggested that a forensic psychiatric service was required for all main courts.

Dr Joseph argued that a large number of psychiatric assessments carried out in prison could still be undertaken by general psychiatrists, especially where the charges were for minor offences. Another contributor suggested that, prior to the recent development of forensic psychiatry, general psychiatrists had carried out such assessments very effectively and efficiently in a city in which he had worked, but liaison was less effective when the doctors had to travel away to other prisons outside their locality. A system in which local psychiatrists could be on hand to see any prisoners in their area would solve this problem.

It was further argued that without a major expansion in forensic psychiatry, general psychiatrists would necessarily be involved with mentally disordered offenders. However, despite effective liaison arrangements with social services departments and general practitioners, there was no similar tradition of establishing relationships with the criminal justice system and there was little appreciation of the scale of the problems involved. Liaison must be widened and the relationship between general and forensic psychiatry carefully considered.

The importance of management and organizational questions for the co-ordination of services was raised. This was a time of high expectations for the effectiveness of management approaches. Despite the relative lack of interest in mentally disordered offenders as a group, there was the possibility of stimulating interest under the banner of management concerns, with which the Home Office and the health, social services and criminal justice agencies were currently preoccupied. More specifically, one contributor suggested that effective liaison could be facilitated by schemes for joint training between the various services. Such schemes were under way with respect to the *Children Act* 1989. Common training materials were being produced for the agencies involved, so that everyone will be aware of what other practitioners need to know.

Dr Wool emphasized the continuing need for effective psychiatric services within the prisons, and for a proper degree of management influence by prison doctors in individual establishments and centrally. In general, the service was 'opening up', with different people coming into the prisons and prison staff working outside. Difficulties in achieving transfers from prison to hospital were highlighted. Concern was expressed about a case in which an inmate had died after being deemed untreatable and unsuitable for transfer. The questioner was particularly disturbed by a judicial ruling concerning another fatality which implied that the standard of hospital care within a prison was not expected to be as high as was required in an outside hospital (*Knight v The Home Office*, 1990). There would always be a need to transfer some individuals from prison to hospital; however, the prisons would increasingly recruit staff to deal with special categories of inmates, such as drug abusers and sex offenders.

The question of resources

A number of contributors discussed ways in which current budgeting arrangements had adverse consequences for the provision of services. Problems arising after the introduction of the 'Fresh Start' working arrangements for prison officers were cited. There was less time available by means of overtime to undertake medical tasks properly. New regulations concerning welfare and housing benefits were also criticized for disadvantaging the homeless and mentally ill. On the other hand, current fiscal concerns had produced unexpected benefits for the probation service. Probation officers were seen as cost effective by the Audit Commission. Some additional money was provided for bail hostels because the probation service could tell a 'good story' about targeting.

There was debate about the cost implications of future developments proposed during the session. Special treatment wings within the prisons, or a possible new psychiatric prison like Grendon Underwood, would be expensive. This was especially the case if these facilities were to match the standards of medical establishments outside the prison service. It was argued that good community care, including the creation of special housing facilities for the homeless mentally ill would be more expensive than current arrangements. There was discussion about the pressure which might be placed by courts on the Treasury to release funds for new services, and it was suggested that the Treasury should be made aware of the cost implications of the current delays occurring within the criminal justice system. Furthermore, schemes such as that described by Dr Joseph required financial resources; more funds were now needed to establish these services more widely. Additional resources were also needed if general psychiatrists were to be persuaded to take on further responsibilities relating to mentally disordered offenders.

By contrast, other contributors argued that new types of provision could result in cost savings in the long run; bail hostel places in Birmingham were two-thirds the cost of hospital places and half the cost of prison places, while a considerable saving to the courts' costs could be made by diverting mentally disordered offenders away from the criminal justice system. Dr Joseph argued that arrangements for diversion should be seen as a switching of resources, rather than as an additional cost. It was claimed that it cost no more to treat mentally disordered offenders properly than to deal with them inappropriately, as at present. However, it was argued that this would still raise the question of from whose budget particular expenditures should be drawn. Solutions may lie in freeing up attitudes to professional boundaries.

Part IV

Planning and implementing new services

12

A view from the private sector

M. LEE-EVANS

Introduction

This paper might have been better entitled: 'A glimpse of the private sector', since I consider myself unable to generalize about provision for mentally abnormal offenders within the private sector as a whole. Instead, I must draw heavily upon my personal experience of the recent expansion of services at Kneesworth House Hospital. Hopefully, this may not prove too limited or biased a sampling of current service provision. The views expressed are essentially my own, and should not be considered to reflect the official views of the management at Kneesworth House Hospital, nor those of the managers of the Psychiatric Division of AMI Healthcare Group plc.[1] I will first consider the context which appears to have created the need and opportunity for the emergence of private sector provision for these patients. Then I will give an account of this provision with specific reference to Kneesworth House Hospital and the functions it has served. Finally, I will take a very tentative look at the future.

The context: 'a right to treatment?'

In contrast with previous legislation, the *Mental Health Act* 1959 can be described as being more utilitarian in seeking to ensure that mentally abnormal offenders should have access to treatment. Although the *Mental Health Act* 1983 has been described as a shift towards legalism, it has preserved and potentially strengthened this utilitarian ideal concerning the disposal of offenders. Thus, Gostin (1983) suggests that part of the current legal approach to psychiatry is the 'ideology of entitlement', i.e. 'that access to health and social services should not be based upon charitable or professional discretion, but upon enforceable rights'.

As Shapland and Williams (1983) have commented, such entitlement begs the issue of the availability and adequacy of treatment services to meet the needs of the abnormal offender. Thus, both Mental Health Acts have also supported the move away from services based upon large institutions, towards community care. As Bluglass commented as early as 1978, the open door policy in local psychiatric hospitals and the transfer of services to district general hospital settings, have resulted in an increasing reluctance to accept difficult patients (Bluglass, 1978). This has created the opportunity for a vicious circle effect, as a lack of experience has compounded a lack of confidence in providing for their needs. As hospital services have become smaller, and as health service personnel are now increasingly prompted to consider the most efficient use of limited resources, one can only anticipate that certain abnormal offenders (particularly those who are not considered sufficiently dangerous for admission to special hospitals), may compete even less successfully for access to conventional psychiatric services (e.g. Coid, 1988a).

The need for special provision for difficult or offender patients who do not require admission to special hospitals has been considered in two government reports. The Glancy Committee considered the need of disturbed patients already within the NHS, who are likely to need secure facilities. It estimated the need for 1000 special beds (DHSS, 1974a). The Butler Committee also considered the plight of the mentally abnormal in the prisons and the community, and established the need for some 2000 secure beds (DHSS, 1974b). This led to a commitment to develop regional secure units to provide 1000 beds in the first instance. However regional health authorities were also prompted to consider the needs for special care units to provide for those patients whose requirements may fall somewhere between ordinary NHS and regional secure unit services. It has been estimated that there were approximately 900 beds available in special units in 1984 (Mason, 1984). A survey conducted by the Forensic Psychiatric Nursing Association in 1988 suggested that some 650 of the proposed 1000 regional secure unit beds had been built. However, only 550 of these were operational.

Quite apart from the apparent shortfall between estimated need and actual provision, there has remained the suspicion that estimates of the potential demand for special facilities have been inadequate (e.g. Royal College of Psychiatrists, 1980). Moreover, there is evidence of an increasing malaise concerning the integration, and therefore the efficiency, of the different services providing secure provision within the NHS (Mental Health Act Commission, 1989). It is in this context that we should consider the actual and potential contribution to this particular client group, from the private sector.

Private sector provision

In England and Wales private psychiatric facilities are formally registered as mental nursing homes under the *Registered Homes Act* 1984. Those which seek to provide for patients detained under mental health legislation, need to be registered additionally for this specific purpose under s.23(3). In its third biennial report, the Mental Health Act Commission (1989) comments on the rapid growth of registered mental nursing homes over recent years, and on the particular difficulties in obtaining reliable information concerning those registered specifically to receive detained patients. Nonetheless, it quotes Department of Health statistics as showing that on 31 March 1988, 63 establishments were registered for this purpose. Although directories of services in the private sector are available (e.g. Laing, 1987; Longman, 1988), this does not allow one to estimate how many beds may be available for detained patients. Nor can one infer the willingness of different establishments to accept detained patients who may have been subject to criminal proceedings, instead of those who may be subject to detention under Part 2 of the *Mental Health Act* 1983. Equally, it is difficult to estimate how many facilities are able to offer a service involving the initial assessment and treatment of mentally abnormal offenders, as opposed to their subsequent rehabilitation or long-term care. However, in general terms, services within the private sector for mentally disordered patients make a significant contribution to long-term care, but a very small contribution to acute care (Connah & Lancaster, 1989; Higgins, 1988). Certainly in commenting on secure provision within the private sector, the Mental Health Act Commission identifies only two sizeable services: the behaviour modification units at St. Andrews Hospital, Northampton, and the services currently provided by AMI at Kneesworth House Hospital and Stockton Hall Hospital (Mental Health Act Commission, 1989). St. Andrews provides a total of 340 beds and a wide spectrum of psychiatric specialties. Although it has been described by the Mental Health Act Commission as providing 'the largest concentration of detained patients outside of the NHS', precise estimates of numbers involved are not given. The Mental Health Act Commission described the services provided by AMI as 'rapidly developing'. Certainly, the service at Kneesworth House Hospital can already lay claim to rivalling many regional secure units in the scope of its provision for abnormal offenders. Combined with its sister hospital at Stockton Hall, it appears poised to become one of the largest providers for abnormal offenders outside of the special hospitals.

Kneesworth House Hospital

The hospital is part of the Psychiatric Division of AMI which provides a total of four units for difficult to place patients.[2] It is situated in 48 acres of grounds in a semi-rural setting approximately 12 miles south-west of Cambridge. It was opened in September 1985 with 49 secure beds for adult mentally disordered patients. In September 1987 it opened an additional 20 beds specifically for mentally handicapped adult patients, and in April 1988 a further 20 beds to provide better opportunities to assess patients in non-secure conditions, prior to transfer to discharge. A further major development is scheduled for completion by September 1990. This is intended to provide a larger range of living units, more adequate patient and staff accommodation and to bring the total comple-ment to 145 beds. The pace of this expansion is made the more striking when one includes the opening of Stockton Hall Hospital, intended to provide a similar service to the North of England with an eventual complement of 54 beds. At the time of writing, 87 of the 89 beds at Kneesworth House were occupied and Stockton Hall is already exceed-ing expectations.

Certain features of the service require discussion to allow an assess-ment of how it relates to provision within the public sector. In discussing these, reference will be made to some preliminary data from a more detailed survey currently being undertaken by Keith Comish, Graham Petrie, Colin Campbell and myself at Kneesworth House. The basic data set relates to a four year, four month period from September 1985 to December 1989. Within this period Kneesworth House received a total of 285 admissions, comprising 245 different patients of whom 32 accounted for 40 re-admissions. Within the same period there were a total of 198 transfers or discharges.

The 'difficult to place' patient

The first point that deserves emphasis is that the service defies most expectations (and even some objections) concerning private sector provi-sion, by providing primarily for patients funded by the public sector rather than for those funded by private insurance or alternative means.

Table 12.1. *Admissions to Kneesworth House Hospital September 1985–December 1989*

Primary reason for admission	Number	%
Physical aggression	183	69.8
Sexual behaviour	19	7.2
Violence//damage to property	12	4.6
Arson	13	5.0
Self-injury	8	3.1
Absconding	8	3.1
Other	19	7.2
Total	262*	100%

* This involves a preliminary analysis involving data from records where the primary presenting problem is clearly recorded.
Note: 23 records require closer examination.

Thus, only three of the 245 patients have not been funded by public services. The vast majority (89%) have been funded by health authorities and the remaining either by social services or by joint health authority and social service funding.

Hitherto, the hospital's policy has been to expand and accommodate its service as far as possible, to those who are experienced as being challenging within the public sector. Only those patients who are too young (less than 16 years), who present serious problems of physical dependency or who would be more appropriately placed in special hospitals, are firmly excluded. Referrals for patients who require very intensive individual treatment programmes are cautiously assessed in the light of existing demands on the service. Otherwise the vast majority of referrals have been accepted.

Although we need to examine our case records in far more detail to obtain a complete picture, the preliminary data presented in Table 12.1 overwhelmingly suggest that it is those patients who present with violence or with some form of physical aggression towards others, who have been difficult to accommodate in the public sector. This appears consistent with descriptions of those patients who are experienced as being challenging within mental handicap services (Emerson *et al.*, 1987). Although the hospital continues to accept the occasional arsonist, child molester or patient likely to present a threat of serious self-injury, the major presenting problem has been the potential threat of aggression or violence towards direct-care staff.

Table 12.2 reveals that the majority of patients are transferred from local hospital settings, with a significant proportion coming directly from the courts. There would appear to be no obvious change in the pattern of the source of admission over time.

However, Table 12.3 clearly reveals a trend towards changes in the legal status of patients. Very few (6%) have recently been admitted as informal patients. The majority of patients remain detained under Part 2 of the *Mental Health Act* 1983, i.e. without becoming involved in criminal proceedings. Nonetheless, there appears a clear trend towards a gradual increase in the proportion of detained patients who have been involved in criminal proceedings. These constituted 40% of all patients admitted during 1988/9. Given that, in the case of mental disorder, the decision to proceed with prosecution may be more arbitrary, (and that violence or physical aggression towards others would normally render one liable to prosecution), the data suggest that the hospital is increasingly providing for a particular client group of mentally disordered people who are potential (if not always actual) offenders.

Length of stay, and disposal

The hospital sets out to prepare patients as quickly as possible for return either to public sector provision or (with the funding authority's agreement) for transfer to alternative long-term private residential care, once sufficient progress is made (Kneesworth House, 1989). To this end, it seeks to provide a specialist acute treatment service and, ideally, would prefer to see most patients transferred within two years of admission. However, it does not exert undue pressure on referrers to remove patients.

The need to justify continued funding, as well as the need to ensure an agreed plan for aftercare, are met by a process of regular review meetings involving the hospital clinical team and professional representatives from funding and (if different) aftercare agencies. These occur six weeks after the patient's admission and every three months subsequently, and involve the submission of written assessment and progress reports. Hitherto, any form of follow-up support or supervision by hospital staff has been rare. More commonly the hospital will facilitate visits from future care-staff to establish rapport with the client and to gain an understanding of his/her needs, before transfer takes place.

Table 12.4 provides a breakdown of the disposal of patients who have left the hospital in the four year, four month period September 1985 to

Table 12.2. *Admissions to Kneesworth House Hospital September 1985–August 1989*

Source of admission over time

From – to	Year 1: Sept '85–Aug '86		Year 2: Sept '86–Aug '87		Year 3: Sept '87–Aug '88		Year 4: Sept '88–Aug '89	
	Number	%	Number	%	Number	%	Number	%
Courts/prison	10	16.4	25	36.0	17	19.3	15	30.0
Special hospital	0	0	1	1.4	3	3.4	1	2.0
NHS hospital	33	54.0	28	41.0	42	47.7	27	54.0
Private sector	7	11.5	5	7.2	7	8.0	2	4.0
Social services	4	6.6	5	7.2	8	9.1	2	4.0
Home	7	11.5	5	7.2	11	12.5	3	6.0
Totals	61	100	69	100	88	100	50	100

Table 12.3. *Admissions to Kneesworth House Hospital September 1985–August 1989*

Legal status

From – to	Year 1: Sept '85–Aug '86		Year 2: Sept '86–Aug '87		Year 3: Sept '87–Aug '88		Year 4: Sept '88–Aug '89	
	Number	%	Number	%	Number	%	Number	%
Informal	15	24.6	10	14.5	29	33.09	3	6.0
Detained Part 2 1983 MHA	33	54.1	39	56.5	32	36.4	27	54.0
Detained Part 3 1983 MHA + CPIA	13	21.3	20	29.0	27	30.6	20	40.0
Totals	61	100	69	100	88	100	50	100

Table 12.4. *Departures from Kneesworth*
House Hospital September 1985–December
1989

Destination	Number	%
Courts/prison	3	2
Special hospital/ISU/RSU	17	6
NHS hospital	73	40
Private sector	38	21
Social services	24	13
Home	33	18
Totals	182	100

Note: This involves a preliminary analysis involving data from discharge records where the departure destination is clearly recorded. Sixteen
records require closer examination.

December 1989. This shows that the vast majority of patients have been
transferred to the public sector, either to local hospital services (43%) or
to local authority provision (16.6%).

Approximately 16% have been discharged to the community and a
further 14% have been transferred to alternative private long-term
residential care. Figure 12.1 reveals that most of the patients who have
left, have been transferred within two years. Indeed it is striking that as
many as 40% have left within three months of admission and 60% have
left within six months. (A possible implication of this finding is discussed
below.)

Figure 12.1 might give one confidence that the service is largely
successful in avoiding the common fear of special units: that beds may
become silted up with long-term patients who cannot be transferred to a
less structured service setting. Indeed, one of the potential criticisms of a
special unit is that it might become a dumping ground and enable
managers to obviate the need for more effort and imaginative initiatives
in treatment and rehabilitation (see Emerson *et al.*, 1987).

However, Fig. 12.2 gives less reason for complacency. Although the
numbers remain small, one can detect a gradually growing longer-term
group. Nonetheless at this stage, this is not too disheartening because
initiatives for the resettlement of most of these longer-term patients are
already well in hand. In many cases they involve more handicapped
patients for whom local services are having to arrange special long-term

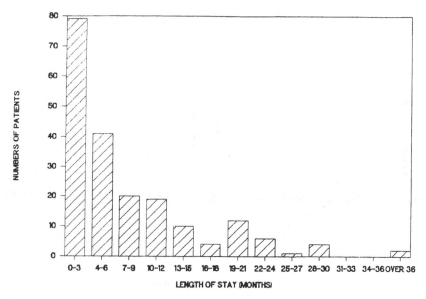

Fig. 12.1. Kneesworth House Hospital departures Sept '85–Dec '89.

provision. In this respect, a more detailed analysis of any changing trends in length of stay should probably take careful account of diagnostic categories.

Key function?

The hospital defines its primary functions in terms of the assessment and treatment of difficult to place patients, and it seeks to provide a conventional range of psychiatric and ancillary services to this end. Whilst these functions are an integral part of the service, it may be that the basic function that the hospital presently serves can be construed as one or other form of crisis intervention. We have yet to complete a detailed analysis of the relationships between sources of admission and subsequent disposal. However, the fact that so many patients have been transferred within three months of admission is the first hint to this effect. Although some acutely disturbed psychotic patients do respond very quickly, it is not plausible to assume that the majority of transfers are taking place because of the demonstration of sudden insights and striking improvements within such a short period of admission. It is more likely

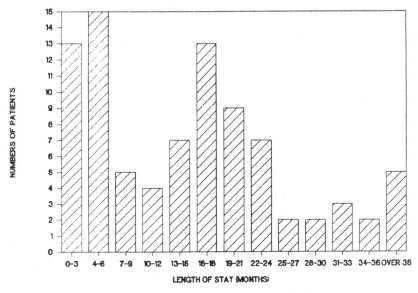

Fig. 12.2. Kneesworth House Hospital resident patients 31/12/89.

that the hospital has provided an important refuge for a public sector service at a time of crisis; a short-term placement enables local services either to resolve the crisis situation or to make arrangements for alternative service provision.

Even when patients do remain for substantially longer periods of assessment and treatment, there may still be a case for seeing the hospital's primary role in terms of crisis intervention. In some cases, local services may simply need more time to plan and provide an alternative service. In other cases, the confidence to make such provision can be boosted by demonstration that patients previously experienced as difficult and frustrating, can in fact show a significant response to a specialized assessment and treatment programme. It must be emphasized that this definition of the hospital's possible real function in terms of crisis intervention, is not intended to denigrate the importance of its assessment and treatment roles. Indeed, to some extent it may even make these slightly more credible, as the service may not need to withstand a more stringent evaluation in terms of demonstrating substantial long-term treatment effects (Emerson *et al.*, 1987). Instead it may be evaluated more fairly in terms of how it enables patients to gain acceptance within less specialized service settings.

The irony will not have escaped the reader that as public sector hospital accommodation is reduced, there is at least one private sector service that is expanding hospital accommodation to meet a consequent need. The disadvantages and dangers of large institutional services are of course at the very basis of arguments for the need for the community care programme. Similarly, cogent arguments have been levelled against special units which attempt to resolve patients' problems in situations remote from those in which the problems have originally presented and to which many patients must return (Emerson *et al.*, 1987). I do not dismiss these disadvantages and dangers and would equally accept the fact that large catchment areas may impede a patient's ability to retain contact with relatives and other potential support within the community (*Mental Health Act Commission*, 1989). These objections must become all the more marked, the more long-term that such provision is allowed to become. However, the present service at Kneesworth House clearly demonstrates that there is a need for a facility to provide some form of crisis intervention function. Moreover, one should not dismiss too quickly the potential advantages of a specialist unit with sufficient resources for the diversification of facilities and the opportunity to accumulate staff expertise and confidence. Ironically, there may even be certain advantages to having such a service provided by the private sector. First, it obviates the need for public services to divert excessive funds away from the community care programme towards establishing special units which would no doubt have reactive effects on local public service provision. Any public service can use the private sector provision if and when required, without any substantial longer-term commitment to that service. Equally, one suspects that the relative speed and ease with which patients are transferred either when alternative services become available for them, or when they have fully graduated from the Kneesworth House programme, may not be entirely unrelated to the cost of funding the Kneesworth placement!

A comment on recent growth

In one sense, the original establishment of Kneesworth House Hospital and its subsequent development must be seen far more as a straightforward consequence of the shortfall in provision in the public sector, rather than the product of any sophisticated market research or aggressive marketing. Indeed, given the possible ambivalence of referrers (i.e. professionals working within the public sector) there was a case for believing that any form of aggressive marketing should be carefully avoided. Neither the establishment of Kneesworth House Hospital nor its subsequent development have been related to any agreements (formal or informal) that it should meet the needs of particular services within the public sector. Its establishment can be traced largely to the entrepreneurship of certain psychiatrists who became aware of the growing number of patients (typically those presenting with violence) who were proving difficult to place in public services. This awareness happily coincided with AMI's readiness to diversify its range of private health services in the British market (Higgins, 1988). The Hospital's subsequent expansion can be seen as the product of a number of factors including:

(a) Proven demand and performance, i.e. its success in filling beds and in meeting budgetary targets.

(b) Its need to establish itself in the market-place as a service that can respond quickly to urgent need. (In this sense full bed-occupancy leading to lengthy waiting lists was to be avoided.)

(c) Its need to rationalize and improve its clinical programme. The final development will involve a total expansion from one to five different units, which will allow for: (i) grouping patients more specifically according to treatment needs, (ii) developing even more specialized assessment and treatment programmes, and (iii) greater variation in security as patients progress.

(d) Finally, of course, there has been the commitment within AMI to the expansion of its Psychiatric Division and the consequent willingness to make the substantial capital investment involved in the establishment of new services.

Towards the future?

Speculating about the future appears a particularly risky exercise given the radical changes in public service provision indicated by the two White Papers: *Working for Patients* and *Caring for People* (Department of Health, 1989*a,b*). Both would seem intended to offer more opportunities and (perhaps even more importantly) to promote more acceptance for public sector usage of private sector services. Both also project the potential for greater competition amongst service providers with the goals of promoting better quality of care and more efficient use of resources.

In theory, at least, there would appear now to be opportunities for the private sector to consider widening its services, either by continuing to provide separate services on a contractual basis, or by entering into joint ventures or even by offering to manage parts of existing public services. Quite apart from extending provision to the existing market (i.e. largely patients who are considered difficult to manage in local hospital services) there may also be an opportunity to extend services to remand patients and to the rehabilitation of special hospital patients. What is evident is that it is certainly not only timely, but now necessary for the private sector to become more pro-active and assertive in marketing its services. In this respect the fact that Kneesworth House Hospital (at a time when it is planning a significant expansion in beds) finds itself in the close vicinity of three of the district health authority services that will be conducting trials with internal markets, appears an interesting coincidence.

However, the prospect of increased competition intended by the White Papers, presupposes the establishment of sufficient service provision to meet possible demand. The services provided by AMI have developed so far not in competition with, but as complementary to, public service provision, because of excess demand on the public sector. Equally, one suspects that the ease with which Kneesworth House has expanded must reflect the lack of any very serious competition for beds within the private sector. Competition that will benefit patients is probably best achieved when there is sufficient supply for the consumer to be allowed choice (Pollitt, 1989).

Given that changes in legislation or clinical practice do not significantly alter the apparent demand for services for abnormal offenders, it is my personal view that a major determinant of future service provision will be staff recruitment. It is in this regard that there is a real danger that the private sector is already, and could become, increasingly drawn into competing with the public sector (Connah & Lancaster, 1989; Owens & Glennerster, 1990). Certainly the difficulty of recruiting staff with sufficient interest and expertise could become a significant barrier to entry for any prospective new services. In this context, one might expect existing services in the private sector to become more actively involved in staff training and development and indeed to seek opportunities for collaboration towards this end.

Discussion

Contributors to the discussion were primarily concerned with understanding how the private sector related to the National Health Service, and how it compared in terms of clinical effectiveness, degree of specialization and relative costs.

The effectiveness of treatments in the private sector

It was pointed out that private hospitals had to be largely self-sufficient; unlike the regional secure units, they could not use other, adjacent psychiatric facilities, and so only limited treatment regimes were available. This limitation could prove a problem for some patients, and it was suggested that private facilities were more suited to the care of chronic patients. It was argued that the ability of the private sector to respond rapidly to problems experienced with patients in other institutions could itself be problematic. The problems of these patients may be very complex, whether they be mentally ill or mentally handicapped, and a mistaken therapeutic decision can prove disastrous. The solution was the setting up of proper National Health Service-based assessment provisions and residential facilities. Mr Lee-Evans argued that the private sector would remain involved in interventionist treatment, but, in direct competition with the National Health Service, it would have to improve and demonstrate its quality of care.

Specialization within the private sector

It was suggested that the private sector had a niche within the overall range of provision for the mentally disordered because it offered some prospect of providing sophisticated assessments and treatments for the apparently untreatable. Faced with the difficulties in dealing with very diverse groups, such as those with various forms of mental impairment who committed different offences, local authorities turned to the private sector. However, it was also suggested that the private sector operated with a short-term model of care, and the question of whether it could expand to cater for the mentally impaired with long-term difficulties was raised. Another contributor pointed out that institutions like Kneesworth House Hospital could organize treatments for these groups because the facility was sufficiently large. However, it was argued that the relationship between the private sector hospitals and other institutions could change if arrangements altered at health district level. The overall context for the development of private sector facilities was described as a change in expectations about the treatment of the mentally disordered. Treatment was now demanded for a broader group than the acutely mentally ill, including substance abusers, aggressive individuals and others with social and psychological problems. In this sense, the health service 'needs' to which the private sector responded were driven by developing expectations.

Mr Lee-Evans responded to this by stating that the private units dealt with a group who obviously required hospitalization; who were seriously mentally impaired or mentally ill. Other facilities were full or would not accept them, and the patients were thus placed in the private sector. Historically, when the private sector in Britain has experienced direct health service competition, one of the first responses has always been to move laterally and to care for those for whom facilities are not being provided, such as the personality disordered. However, this strategy did not mean that attempts would not continue to be made to improve the clinical effectiveness of the services the private sector provided. Being market-led maintains a positive, task orientated attitude among staff working in the private sector (and also tends to minimize the professional demarcation disputes and prolonged agonizing discussions which can sometimes characterize the health service). Mr Lee-Evans considered that one possible future direction was the setting up of supported facilities closer to the community so that individuals did not inappropriately remain in the acute hospital setting.

The cost effectiveness of the private sector

Questions were raised about the development of the private sector in the context of the financial stringencies facing health authorities. It was pointed out that the group of patients being considered for placement were, in any event, a very expensive group to care for. It was suggested that one reason why the health service turns to the private sector might be that the present regional model for forensic services is not appropriate. The private hospitals take patients from anywhere in the country. It was further suggested that resources may be misplaced within the regions: with better internal communication, patients may be treatable within the health service and more cheaply than in the private sector. Another contributor argued that the private hospitals were cost effective, not in competition with the regional secure units, but with general psychiatric units in local psychiatric hospitals and district general hospitals, where the establishment and maintenance of small special units would be more expensive than funding private placements. Thus the private sector dealt with problems arising at the district level, and its niche was really challenging patients who were not appropriate for a regional secure unit placement.

A question was raised about relative pay levels in the two sectors, both for consultants and for nursing staff. One contributor pointed out that non-professional staff were more widely used in the private hospitals than in the regional secure units. In reply it was suggested that pay in the private sector varied, but some professionals were paid more than in the health service. The competition was really for nurses, rather than for other staff, but people moved into the service for reasons other than remuneration. The lack of inter-professional disputes could be one reason why a move was attractive. However, jobs were less secure in the private sector, with services being market-led, although it was this need to maintain a market edge which contributed to the positive professional feeling within the private sector.

Possible changes in the financial circumstances affecting the private sector were referred to. It was pointed out that, with the advent of the reforms in the structure of the NHS (Department of Health, 1989*b*), district health authorities might find that it would become worthwhile to attract patients, and hence funds, from other districts into special facilities set up to care for mentally disordered offenders. It was argued that one response to the need to contain financial commitments to individuals at the local level was for special funds to follow the most difficult patients into local facilities, perhaps with a premium from the Home Office, thus allowing general psychiatry to respond to the special needs of these groups.

Mr Lee-Evans suggested that the private sector would respond to changes within health service arrangements by becoming more competitive. At the moment, there were instances when health authorities wanted to keep patients at facilities like Kneesworth House because it was cheaper than providing care locally, and this occurred despite the clinical judgement that the patient would now be better placed elsewhere. However, these problems were not so severe as those experienced by the special hospitals because the health authorities save expenditure of substantial sums of money when patients move out of the private sector and back into the care of district services.

Notes

1. Kneesworth House Hospital was originally established by American Medical International Hospitals Limited, part of American Medical

International Inc. In February 1988 the company was floated on the British Stock Exchange as AMI Healthcare Group plc.
2. Apart from Kneesworth House and Stockton Hall Hospitals, the Psychiatric Division also provides 36 beds for adolescents and young people at Langton House, Swanage, and an 18 bed head injury rehabilitation unit at Grafton Manor, Northampton.

13

Case management

G. SHEPHERD

Introduction

The long-term mentally ill have much in common with mentally disordered offenders. Apart from some direct overlap, both groups have similar long-term needs across a wide range of problem areas (psychiatric, psychological, social, occupational, etc) and these needs can only be met by co-operation between a number of different agencies (health, social services, housing, voluntary bodies, etc). Both groups may also spend periods of time away from normal society and therefore face problems of social re-integration and the transition between segregated and open settings. It is therefore instructive to examine issues concerned with the future pattern of provision for mentally abnormal offenders from the perspective of our experience with the long-term mentally ill.

In most countries the pattern of services for people with long-term mental illness has changed dramatically over the past 25 years. There has been a concerted effort to shift the location and organization of care away from large, remote, and old-fashioned mental hospitals towards smaller, more community-based mental health services. The extent to which this shift in the pattern of service provision has been successfully achieved varies greatly both within and between particular countries, but there is now fairly good evidence that if community services are properly planned and properly targeted on those in greatest need then it is possible to produce a pattern of community-based provision which benefits the majority of those with long-term psychiatric and social needs (Bachrach & Lamb, 1989; Thornicroft & Bebbington, 1989). From a policy point of view, the main lesson that has emerged from this process is that it is very much easier to set a goal which involves the elimination of a particular kind of institutional provision (the mental hospital) than it is to put an effective alternative in its place. The lack of effective alternatives to replace the mental hospital is partly due to lack of resources, but it is also partly attributable to a lack of agreement over what might constitute a comprehensive range of service provisions appropriate to a specific set of local conditions and priorities.

One element of service that most people would agree is crucial to the effective functioning of a community-based mental health service is a mechanism for co-ordinating and maintaining continuity of care. Within the traditional institution, co-ordination, monitoring, and continuity of care were provided, to use Goffman's famous phrase, 'under one roof and one authority' (Goffman, 1961) and even then standards could leave a lot to be desired. The attempt to break up the total institution, to disperse care, and to provide it from many different sites, and under many different authorities, thus raises the immediate problem of how to glue services back together again and achieve an integrated and continuous service built around individual needs. One possible solution which has emerged to this problem is known as case management.

Case management may therefore be seen as an inevitable consequence of the move towards more community-based patterns of service and, if the recent White Paper on community care is to be taken at face value, case management will form the cornerstone of community care in the future (Department of Health, 1989a). What I intend to do in this paper is to examine the concept of case management and some of its advantages and disadvantages. Throughout my discussion I will try to relate back to the problems of service provision for the mentally disordered offender, although our experience of case management – such as it is – is firmly rooted in the care of non-offender patients. It must also be acknowledged that case management represents the latest in a long line of magic solutions to hit community psychiatry. Like many good ideas it risks being oversold and then rejected as people become disillusioned because it has failed to live up to its promises. Case management, as we shall see, is not a panacea; it is a useful idea which addresses a central problem to do with the co-ordination and monitoring of community services. It is not a substitute for an adequate range of community provisions.

What is case management?

Our current concepts of case management depend very much on experience in the United States. The classic description of the elements of a case management approach is to be found in Intagliata (1982). He lists five main components:

(*a*) A comprehensive assessment of individual needs.
(*b*) The development of an individualized package of care to meet those needs.
(*c*) Ensuring that the individual gains access to these services. This may entail considerable outreach work, i.e. going along with the client to the housing, or social security office, or day centre to ensure that they are able to actually obtain whatever service they need and that it conforms, as far as possible, to their expressed wishes and desires. There is thus an additional element which lays emphasis on the value of consumer choice in determining service provision.
(*d*) Monitoring the quality of services provided and liaising with service providers if the quality or content of services does not meet what is required and, if necessary, attempting to change them, i.e. case managers may be proactive in actually changing and shaping services.
(*e*) Offering long-term, flexible support, adjusted according to fluctuating levels of individual need.

The underlying concept is thus of one agency, usually presumed to be a single individual, who has a clearly defined responsibility to provide individualized, long-term care, in a flexible and sensitive manner. The case manager co-ordinates the inputs of a number of different agencies, provides consistency and commitment, and acts as an advocate on behalf of the client (and their family) to ensure that they receive the right package of services. He/she also monitors the quality of services provided and ensures that continuity is maintained over time. The concept is clear enough, but it contains a number of tensions and ambiguities.

First, is the primary responsibility of the case manager to the client, or to the system? Should the case manager be primarily concerned with the efficient use of resources, or with the creation of a high-quality, individually tailored, service? Of course, the answer is that, in the best of all worlds, the two should not be in conflict. However, in the real world they may be, and this tension may cause problems. Some kind of balance must be struck between these two competing demands of individual need and economic efficiency, but we must recognize the danger that case management could be a mechanism for exerting even tighter control over resources, and this danger is also present for the mentally disordered offender. We are all familiar with innovations that have been highly appealing on clinical grounds, but have been exploited, even corrupted, by economic considerations.

Secondly, how are case managers meant to operate? Are they simply there to link up clients to services in a rather bureaucratic, administrative way, as a kind of agency broker, or, should they use their relationship with the client as a special kind of therapeutic support? The former corresponds to a managerial concept of case management, the latter to a more clinical, casework model. Clearly, it is the latter model which is more like the traditional role of the experienced probation officer or forensic psychiatrist who provides long-term support and advice for the offender patient. There is little empirical evidence which would allow one to assess just how important this relationship aspect of case management might be. However, Gunn and Taylor note that:

As far as offending behaviour is concerned, one of the few factors which has been demonstrated to be effective in prevention is a supportive relationship with a relative, friend, or professional adviser.

(Gunn & Taylor, 1983: p. 116)

Regarding the long-term mentally ill, Harris and Bergman (1987) argue that case managers should consciously cultivate the therapeutic aspects of their relationships with clients to help them deal more effectively with their problems. Case managers can help clients integrate their functioning, act as a sounding board to help them develop a better, more reliable, sense of reality, improve their problem-solving skills, etc. At the heart of this process is a stable, consistent relationship. Of course, in most situations both managerial and clinical elements of case management will be present simultaneously, but funding agencies must be clear as to exactly what kind of case management service they expect as this has both training and resource implications, as discussed below.

Who should act as case manager?

Depending upon what concept of case management one favours, there are different implications regarding who is most suitable to act as a case manager. If one favours a simple, managerial model, then case managers may be recruited from relatively inexperienced, non-professional staff. If one favours a more clinical model, then one would require experienced, highly trained (and well-supervised) clinicians. The two models therefore also have very different funding implications. In the context of the

National Health Service, the question of who should function as case manager is complicated since the role combines elements of many different mental health professions – social work, nursing, psychiatry, clinical psychology, even occupational therapy. There have even been suggestions to invent a new profession, but this does not seem very practical. In the White Paper, the Government states that it 'does not wish to be prescriptive about the background from which the case manager should be drawn' (Department of Health, 1989a). This may be a wise stance, but does not help us very much in the resolution of these difficult inter-professional issues. Because of the overlap between professional roles, whoever does take on the role of case manager may thus meet considerable resistance from their colleagues. If case managers are to function effectively, then these issues will have to be addressed. Case managers cannot be held responsible for the provision of services unless other service providers are willing to co-operate. In the context of services for offenders, the added complications of medico-legal and other statutory requirements may restrict the range of options of those who might take on full case management responsibilities.

What training will case managers require?

It is clear from everything that has been said so far that, in order to implement case management systems effectively, a considerable input of new training will be required. However, it is not clear exactly what this training should contain. As indicated earlier, case management is predicated on a careful assessment of individual needs but, as yet, there is little agreement on how this should be done. The technical problems involved in assessing needs for care amongst long-term psychiatric patients in the community are extremely complex and there are some very difficult underlying conceptual and methodological issues (see Brewin *et al.*, 1987; Brewin & Wing, 1988; Brugha *et al.*, 1988). To determine whether or not a need for service is present implies not only being able to decide whether or not some problem or difficulty is present, but also whether or not some potentially effective intervention (service) exists to remedy it. Both decisions demand considerable value judgements and whether they can be made reliably and validly remains doubtful. The development of suitable instruments to assess need, and appropriate training packages to use them, is therefore an urgent priority.

The White Paper suggests that the procedure for assessment of needs should be left to the discretion of individual local authorities and that it should be carried out simply, informally and timeously (Department of Health, 1989*a*). It also suggests that 'all agencies and professions involved with the individual and his or her problems should be brought into the assessment procedure when necessary' and goes on to list seven lines of potential contributors. How to reconcile these two pieces of advice will no doubt be made clear when the detailed codes of guidance are issued in due course. The question of training and technical support is particularly important if the responsibility is going to fall mainly onto social workers since they have come under criticism in recent years because of the alleged loss of specialist expertise and the inadequacy of their training for working with the mentally ill (House of Commons, 1985: paras 200–201). Similar arguments would apply if social service departments were to be charged with the responsibility of assessing the needs of mentally disordered offenders.

Apart from the technical aspects of training, there are also important conceptual issues that need to be taken into account when thinking of the training needs of case managers. Chronic patients are generally seen as unattractive to work with, they are often difficult to motivate, they may be unco-operative, unwilling, or unable to try new experiences and activities, they may be abusive, even physically violent. They are certainly seldom top of the popularity ratings among therapeutically ambitious young professionals who see their primary role as treating people and making them better. In all these respects, the long-term mentally ill share much in common with many mentally disordered offenders and one of the most important elements in the training of case managers to work with either group will therefore be good support and supervision from experienced, and high status, practitioners in the field. It has been suggested that the failure to provide this kind of support in the past contributed to the tendency of community services to drift upmarket away from the most difficult patients and towards less demanding, more tractable customers. If this trend is not to be repeated with case management services, then it requires not only monitoring and supervision, but also good leadership and emotional support.

Case management and the problems of working together

Case management is not a magic solution to the problems of inter-agency collaboration or multi-disciplinary teamwork; it will simply move them to a different context. In an interesting paper, Meuller and Hopp (1987) describe the attitudinal, administrative, legal and financial problems that they encountered in trying to set up a case management system for patients being discharged from a state hospital. In particular, they focus on problems of inter-agency collaboration. From their experience, it is quite clear that case management does not eradicate the suspicion and rivalry which often characterizes the relationship between caring agencies; indeed, it may make them worse. This situation is likely to be compounded in the UK since the proposals in the new White Paper (Department of Health, 1989*a*) which seek to clarify the responsibilities between health and social services in the care of the long-term mentally ill may well simply accentuate their differences. Case managers may then be caught in the middle. To sustain joint working means retaining joint planning and being prepared to continue working at the difficult and time consuming task of inter-agency collaboration. The problems will be as great – or even greater – when it comes to maintaining joint working relationships between health services, probation services, and the prisons.

Even within a single agency, case managers will still have to wrestle with the familiar problems of multi-disciplinary teamwork since, as we noted earlier, some degree of teamwork is inevitable in order to resolve basic questions of professional accountability. Case managers cannot do everything by themselves; their role is to co-ordinate a number of different inputs and a crucial part of their skills is to recognize what they cannot be held responsible for, as well as what they can do, and then to ensure that their colleagues discharge their agreed responsibilities with respect to each individual case. There is even a view that case management is best seen as a team responsibility (Test, 1979). She argues that, providing teams are clear about their responsibilities on a day-to-day basis, they may come to better decisions than individuals, are less vulnerable to sickness and holidays, and provide better protection against burnout. It must be said that these propositions have yet to be experimentally tested.

Probably the most important area for case managers in terms of inter-agency co-operation concerns the transition of patients in and out of hospital. In the last few years there have been a number of reports of radical community-based programmes which aim to prevent, or at least minimize, in-patient admission for people experiencing acute psychiatric crises (e.g. Stein & Test, 1985; Hoult, 1986). Similar projects are currently being conducted in this country. The results from these programmes suggest that, although there are some advantages in trying to treat patients as far as possible in the community, particularly in terms of their social recovery, even the most aggressive forms of community-based treatment do not remove the need for admission entirely. They can significantly reduce lengths of admission – and thereby markedly reduce costs – but treatment in the community is not a substitute for treatment in hospital, it is complementary to it. Even with the best community-based care there will still be a need to co-ordinate the activities of hospital-based and community-based practitioners. Similar boundary disputes between different agencies are also common in the care of mentally disordered offenders and case managers will not make them suddenly disappear.

Is case management effective?

This may seem like the most important question of all but, as is often the case, there is only very limited evidence regarding the effectiveness of case management systems (Anthony *et al.*, 1988; Fisher *et al.*, 1988). Much of the evidence is inconclusive or somewhat contradictory, but there are two good quality controlled trials. Bond *et al.* (1988) working in Indiana, describe a random controlled trial evaluating assertive case management (ACM) across three different urban community mental health centres (CHMCs). In each centre, subjects were randomly assigned to either ACM, or the standard programme, and 167 subjects were evaluated in total across a range of outcome criteria. Data were only available for the first six months of the project, but by this time subjects receiving ACM were showing significantly fewer admissions and less time in hospital than controls and this resulted in significant savings in costs. There were no other significant differences. The authors comment that this may be a reflection of the relatively short time scale of the study. The results were particularly interesting in that the ACM package seemed to work very well in two of the centres, however, in the third, ACM actually did significantly worse than the control condition. Bond *et al.* discuss some of the possible reasons for this, e.g. sample differences, lack of clarity over the programme's aims, and the presence of a powerful conflicting ideology.

Goering *et al.* (1988) working in Toronto, followed up matched groups of patients (*n* = 82 in each group) comparing those provided with a trained case manager with those receiving traditional aftercare without intensive, personalized support. After six months there were few differences between the two groups. However, by two years the case management group showed superior outcomes on a range of occupational and social measures. The authors note that their results support the value of case managers, but underline the need to allow adequate time before evaluating their impact. They also note that case management appeared to have little effect on rates of rehospitalization. They attribute this mainly to 'the limited influence of case managers on the control of patients' medical and other kinds of therapeutic care.'

These two papers therefore provide complementary pictures of the effectiveness of case management systems. Bond *et al.* succeeded in reducing rehospitalization over six months, but failed to improve functioning. Goering *et al.* succeeded in improving functioning over a two year period, but failed to affect rehospitalization. Taken together, the studies underline the need to allow adequate time for the evaluation of the effects of case management and also the potential specificity of local conditions. A major difference between the two studies lies in the degree to which the case managers were integrated into the clinical teams who were responsible for monitoring the patients' symptoms and taking decisions about whether or not to admit to hospital. In the case of Bond *et al.* they were fully involved; in the case of Goering *et al.* they were not. This probably accounts for the failure to affect re-hospitalization rates in the latter study. Thus, if case management is to be effective in improving functioning and keeping people out of hospital, case managers need to be able to influence both the psychiatric and the social aspects of people's problems. This has clear implications for the kinds of organizational links that are necessary in order for case managers to function effectively. If they are not properly integrated into the existing network of services, then they are going to find their jobs extremely difficult. Once again, this underlines the potential difficulties of creating too sharp a split between health and social forms of care as envisaged in the White Paper (Department of Health, 1989*a*).

Conclusions

The need for some kind of system to co-ordinate services for people with long-term mental illness stems directly from policies aimed at de-institutionalizing large numbers of chronically mentally ill people. Unless active steps are taken, patients may receive even worse care and some-times no care at all – in the community compared with hospital. Mentally disordered offenders, like the long-term mentally ill, need individualized packages of care from a number of different agencies and dispersed across a number of different sites. Case management is a possible solution to these problems, but it can never be a substitute for services themselves.

There are great dangers that service providers will place too much emphasis on the development of case management and too little on the service infrastructure on which the work of the case managers depends. If we are to move away from services that rely on the mental hospital then we must first aim to reprovide the full range of functions that the hospitals provided (housing, medical care, occupation, social support, etc) from a community base. Then, and only then, do we need sophisticated case management systems. As far as the mentally disordered offender is concerned, they will also require access to a similarly comprehensive range of services. Case management may be one element in this range of provision, perhaps a particularly useful one, but no more than that.

Discussion

The discussion of case management focused on questions of effectiveness, cost and confidentiality.

The effectiveness of case management

The role of non-professionals and voluntary workers was considered. Within the social services, case management systems were designed to enable social work professionals to co-ordinate the work of non-professionals. Facilities for the homeless, for example, were sometimes largely staffed by non-professionals. The co-ordination and supervision of services provided by non-professionals was a time-consuming exercise. This should be recognized in any appraisal of the effectiveness of the case management approach. In contrast, reference was made to the work of the Elmore Committee for patients within the Oxford area who proved 'difficult to place' with care agencies, and where something like a case management approach had been initiated by non-professionals to secure care agreements for the clients (Vagg, 1987). Concern was voiced by another contributor about this research. By re-labelling individuals 'difficult to place' rather than 'difficult', a more positive attitude towards them had been generated. However, these people were difficult to place because they were difficult; abusing drugs and alcohol or being assaultive, for example. The success of the scheme was secured through a sleight of hand, and it was possible that case managers more generally might become involved in a whole series of complex and dubious negotiations on behalf of clients. What is needed is a more direct acknowledgement of the qualities and needs of these clients by case managers and care agencies. A more specific question was raised about the relation of the case manager to the courts. This would have to be clearly defined if the approach was to prove successful for the care in the community of mentally disordered offenders.

Dr Shepherd referred to experience in the United States where case managers had control of funds for clients. This control of case budgets was one mechanism through which the case manager might be able to negotiate effectively and openly for clients.

Budgeting for the case management approach

The theme of budgetary arrangements was taken up by other contributors. One emphasized that the only effective way for the approach to be funded was for the case manager to have access to his or her own specific budget, or for funds to be linked to particular clients. It was argued that a simple supply and demand model for the market for care services could not be applied. The agencies responded to effective demand, but clients did not demand the services they required, hence the role of the case manager. Dr Shepherd commented that he had avoided the complex question of resources in his paper, but the relation of case management to budgetary arrangements was important, although whether it was best to devolve budgets right down to the case level was not yet established.

Confidentiality of records

The difficulty was raised of defining and controlling who had access to client records when care was provided on an inter-agency basis. Records of case management assessments and reviews would have to be kept. There was always a problem when a variety of professional groups were involved. Should there be an integrated 'replacement' system of records, or should the agencies keep different sets of records in parallel? The technical question of access to computerized records was simple to solve; it was easy to provide different levels of access based on a system of passwords. More difficult was the question of who should have access at these different levels, a problem to which there was no easy solution, and which had to be considered in local steering committees.

14

A view from the Department of Health

J. REED

Policy for mental health services in England is based on two straight-forward principles. These are first, that care should be provided as locally to where a person lives as is reasonably possible, and secondly, that treatment should be available in the least restrictive conditions that are compatible with the safety of the patient, of those looking after him and of the public at large. In considering the practical application of these principles, I make no apology for reviewing the history of policy and practice; it is not possible, in my view, to understand the mental health services we are trying to achieve for the future without understanding how the service has developed over the years. I do so, against a background of the radical changes that have occurred in the provision of services for mentally ill and mentally impaired patients generally, in criminal justice legislation and in the judicial process; and, perhaps most importantly, in public perceptions and attitudes. An evaluation of the extent of the implications of these developments, and the impact that they have had specifically on the nation's response to the needs of the mentally disordered offender is, I would suggest, at the heart of our business here today.

When examining a service it is easy to sound over-critical. We must not forget that, in general, hospital services for mentally disordered people have improved out of all recognition in the last 30 years. You only have to read the review of developments published by the Hospital Advisory Service in 1985 to see the fundamental changes for the better that have taken place. Rereading the reports of 1969 about Ely Hospital and 1972 about Whittingham Hospital shows how services have improved (HMSO, 1969, 1972). Even the time that I have been in psychiatry has seen the disappearance of wards of 40 people, heated by a single coal fire in winter. In those days, outbreaks of paratyphoid were common and death frequent. The reports to the Board of Control up to 1959, when I first worked in general psychiatry, speak of severe staff shortages – nurses and doctors were almost impossible to recruit. In 1949, there were 405 consultant psychiatrists. In 1987, there were 1924 and some 3500 other medical staff. In 1961, there were six consultants in the special hospitals; in 1986 there were 33. Out-patient clinics were a novelty in 1959. There was virtually no community support and the rule of thumb given to a newcomer was admit the patient first and think about it later. The large hospital system was no golden age for patients, though the medical superintendent carved my lunch each day in person and my car was cleaned three times a week – free!

I will start at the beginning, with the early organization of services. The idea of a local service is by no means new. Before the Elizabethan Poor Laws, abbeys and monasteries provided what care there was as a religious duty. The *Poor Law Act* of 1601 and the *Settlement Act* of 1661 firmly tied services to the local community, making the parish responsible for the funding and provision of care.

It is not unreasonable to view the development of non-local services in the 19th century as being an abnormal phenomenon in the long-standing pattern of local mental health care. The *Asylum Act* 1808 gave local authorities permissive power to build mental hospitals and the *Lunatic Asylum Act* 1845 obliged authorities, within three years, to provide hospitals, usually on a county basis. However, no sooner is the asylum system actively developing than we see the first moves away from it.

The first domiciliary Crisis Intervention Service was set up in the 1880s. In 1889, the first out-patient clinic was started. In 1918, the Board of Control suggested that early treatment units in general hospitals would be helpful in speeding recovery. This movement back towards local care is reflected in the Mental Treatment Act 1930 which, among other things, allowed treatment without certification. As is usual in the mental health field, policy developments reflected, rather than led, improvements in clinical practice and, particularly, the realization that better results could often be obtained with less reliance on in-patient care and a greater use of out-patient and domiciliary care.

It was against this setting that the major tranquillizers were introduced in the mid-1950s. The effect of these combined events was dramatic. On 31 December 1954 there were 152 197 patients in mental illness hospitals and units in England and Wales. By 1969 there were just over 116 000 and at the end of 1986 there were some 60 000. These changes in hospital population and clinical practice commanded great interest at the Ministry of Health, as it was then, not least through the influential paper by Tooth and Brooke setting out the changes in the hospital population to date and predicting a further decline in hospital population to levels very near the present one (Tooth & Brooke, 1961).

The policy consequences of these changes was first set out in Enoch Powell's famous 'Water Towers' speech given to the MIND Annual General Meeting in March 1961. This was the first statement of a policy that governments of both parties have since pursued steadily. The basic requirement of this policy is that health authorities should develop comprehensive services both for mentally ill and for mentally handicapped people and that this should be done in association with local authorities and voluntary organizations. This policy was set out in detail in the White Papers, *Better Services for Mentally Handicapped* (DHSS, 1971*b*) and *Better Services for Mentally Ill* (DHSS, 1975), and so far as mental illness is concerned has, most recently, been restated in outline by the Parliamentary Secretary for Health, Roger Freeman, in his statement of Mental Illness Initiatives in association with the Government's Response to the Griffiths' Report in July 1989.

Turning now to the particular group of patients who are the concern of this conference and who have been the focus of much inquiry and research over the years. The report of a Select Committee of the House of Commons quoted research showing some 1900 mentally disordered people to be inappropriately housed in non-asylum secure accommodation. The Select Committee reported that the conditions in which the patients were held were 'revolting' and recommended the establishment of regional secure hospitals. That was in 1807. The Select Committee report led directly to the development of the mental hospital system. Coming now to more recent times, all relevant policy statements, even those as early as Enoch Powell's 'Water Towers' speech, have recognized the need for some patients to be treated in conditions of security. This need has not always been met. Although this failure is commonly ascribed to lack of beds, even in years when many more mental illness and mental handicap beds existed, similar problems occurred. This is clear from the setting up by the Department of Health in January 1971 of a working party to review existing guidance on security in NHS hospitals (which, of course, at that time excluded the special hospitals), to consider the present and future needs of such security and to make recommendations. This committee – the eponymous Glancy Committee – produced a report in July 1973 which was circulated as a discussion paper. Its final report was produced in March 1974 (DHSS, 1974*a*).

Somewhat later, in September 1972, the Butler Committee was established jointly by the Department of Health and the Home Office. The second of Butler's terms of reference was 'to consider what, if any, changes are necessary in powers, procedures and facilities for the provision of appropriate treatment in prison, hospital or the community for offenders suffering from mental disorder'. The Butler Committee produced an interim report in July 1974 and a final report in 1975 (DHSS, 1974*b*; Home Office & DHSS, 1975). The Glancy Committee, reviewing the position in the early 1970s, found a mismatch between needs and resources though not, as you might assume, one due to a shortage of beds (DHSS, 1974*a*). Having been set up because of an apparent lack of secure beds in NHS, they found that in 1971 there were, in psychiatric hospitals, some 13 000 beds in wards which were regularly locked by day, which included severely subnormal, elderly and general psychiatric patients. They considered however, that the great majority of these beds were being used for secure treatment, when other arrangements would have been more appropriate. Patients were in these wards either from force of therapeutic habit or through shortage of staff, and Glancy considered that the great majority of the patients could be treated in more open conditions. However, they estimated that some 1000 patients currently in NHS hospitals needed treatment in conditions of more security than was available. These 1000 beds, Glancy recommended, should be provided in regional secure units. The Butler Committee, in its interim report, strongly supported the creation of regional secure units. It was proposed that, if account was also taken of patients needing treatment in conditions of security below the level provided in the special hospitals but who currently were not in NHS care, then 2000 beds would be necessary.

The need for regional secure units was accepted by the then Secretary of State Mrs Barbara Castle, and both capital and revenue made available for the development and running both of interim units and of the established units to the level of 1000 beds, i.e. 20 beds per million of population in the first instance, but Mrs Castle indicated that there should be a reconsideration of the position in light of experience of the new system.

Significant progress has also been made in mental health legislation relating to mentally disordered offenders. The Butler Committee made recommendations for the reform of legislation for this group – and some of these are found in the *Mental Health Act* 1983, Part III. As you know, courts may now remand mentally disordered offenders to hospital for a medical report, remand to hospital for treatment and also make interim hospital orders. Whether or not the courts have taken anything like sufficient advantage of these provisions is debatable, and this is something that is being actively pursued by my ministers and their Home Office colleagues.

More recently, the most important development has been the decision by ministers to move the management of the special hospitals from the Department of Health to a new special health authority. The move arose because of increasing concern, within the Department and elsewhere, at the Special Hospital Service's professional and organizational isolation. Also, there was a growing awareness that the hospitals were not receiving the benefits of general management either locally or centrally, and we acknowledge that the Department of Health as a department of state simply did not have the specialist skills of hospital management that are essential to the running of a modern cost-effective Health Service. The new Special Hospital Service Authority was established on 1 July 1989 and took over the running of the hospitals from the Department of Health on 1 October 1989.

So much then for the policy and provision background to the health care of the mentally disordered offender. How effectively has this been translated into bricks and mortar and personnel? Problems in developing secure treatment facilities are nothing new. An early secure unit became operational at 27% over capital budget. That was at Bedlam in 1814. Regional variation in service provision is not a new phenomenon either – in 1714 Croydon was one of only three places in England that refused to admit the mentally ill to its almshouses.

Special hospitals

There are at present some 1700 beds within the Special Hospital Service on the three campuses and we are confident that the new management arrangements will lead to very real benefits to those patients who need treatment in conditions of special security. They already make a significant contribution in meeting the needs of the mentally disordered offender 15% of all those placed on hospital orders are treated in special hospitals. However, we are mindful of research such as that done by Dell and Robertson which suggests that of the sample of mentally ill male patients in Broadmoor whom they saw, only 28% needed the degree of security that was available there and nearly 50% were rated as definitely or probably suitable for treatment in conditions of lesser security (Dell & Robertson, 1988). Yet transfer is not always easy to achieve. In

December 1988, we knew of 47 patients in special hospitals who had been recommended for a move to another hospital on trial leave or transfer, but were awaiting a vacancy. Of these, four had been waiting for between one and two years and two for between two and three years.

Additionally, we have the report of the Health Advisory Service on its visit to Broadmoor Hospital which clearly indicates the considerable tasks facing the hospital, the Special Hospital Service Authority and the Department of Health in bringing the hospital up to acceptable modern standards (NHS Health Advisory Service/DHSS Social Services Inspectorate, 1988).

Ministers have also provided the new Authority with a set of policy guidelines that seek to relate these broad aims to the future development of the service. In a wide-ranging review such as this it would be inappropriate for me to go into any greater detail. But it may be instructive to note that, amongst the issues highlighted in that paper is the essential need to view special hospital provision as an integral component of the wider spectrum of psychiatric provision, and to develop much more effective working links between all of the agencies concerned.

Regional secure units

All regions bar one have a regional secure unit treating mentally ill and psychopathically disordered patients in conditions of medium security. One region has a secure unit for mentally handicapped people and another has a secure unit for adolescents. There are, overall, 530 beds and approximately a further 180 are planned. Regional secure units (RSUs) were established with the remit of keeping people for a maximum of two years. In setting this target level for RSU provision it is clear that the Glancy Committee had a different view of the function of special hospitals from that which obtains today. The Glancy Committee considered that patients who were not well enough to move to less secure accommodation after 18 months to two years in an RSU could reasonably be moved on to a special hospital for long-term care. This does not accord with the present views that the function of a special hospital is to provide treatment only when special security is needed and that they should not be used for long-term care of patients needing a lesser degree of security. Despite the recommendation for 1000 beds from Glancy and 2000 from Butler, we actually have just over 500 – only a quarter of those recommended by Butler. It seems clear that not all the money allocated to the regional secure unit programme has been spent by health authorities in the way that was intended. Between 1976–77 and 1981–82 DHSS allocated £44¼ million revenue for the development and operation of RSU and interim secure units. Of this amount nearly £18m was spent on security in psychiatric hospitals, £14¼m on other psychiatric services and some £12m was spent elsewhere in the NHS (Hansard, 6 December 1982: 389–391).

The general psychiatric services

Facilities for treatment in conditions of security below that of an RSU but above that of an open ward are reported to be fairly widely available in the psychiatric services nationally. The last return in 1986 showed that there were 868 beds in wards which were permanently locked and 308 in beds which were sometimes locked. This represents an average of just over five beds per district health authority, although some districts have none. There were, in addition, 785 beds in locked wards in mental handicap hospitals or four per health authority. There was within the Glancy Report an implicit recommendation that the many inappropriately locked beds in the mental hospitals should be opened (DHSS, 1974a). With the fall in secure beds in mental hospitals from some 13 000 to the present 2000 it is clear that the implicit recommendation has been acted on, perhaps more effectively and expeditiously than the explicit recommendation for the development of RSUs.

The forensic psychiatric services in the form of special hospitals and RSUs, are not separate from the rest of the general psychiatric services. It is important to remember that, when they are ready, patients will move back to district facilities and the community. Indeed, most mentally disordered offenders can be appropriately cared for in a local setting and in conditions of minimal security. The message must be that services should be available in the right place and at the right time.

The private sector

The Health Service makes use of the facilities provided by the private sector for some particular clinical groups. For some particular geographic areas, this can amount to a very considerable financial commitment and may reflect the success of the private sector in identifying gaps in present provision and responding to these more rapidly than the state sector. Time does not permit any discussion of the accompanying growth in numbers of personnel who support these hospital services.

The passage of time since the Glancy and the Butler Reports has seen many changes in the mental health service and a considerable development in what is achievable in mental health care. Despite all these changes, I cannot say that all is as I would wish in the present stage of forensic psychiatric services in England. At the level of individual cases we are aware of difficulty in providing long-term treatment in conditions of medium security for all categories of disorder, of treatment in medium security for mentally handicapped people and of the difficulties presented to the criminal justice system by these deficiencies and by problems in obtaining speedy and effective intervention by the Health Service in diverting or removing mentally disordered offenders from the criminal justice system. Health authorities need to plan for a flexible range of secure facilities, tailored to their patients' requirements. A regional forensic psychiatry service is wholly fulfilling its function only when no special hospital patients or mentally disordered prisoners assessed as appropriate for transfer experience long delays in finding suitable regional facilities to move to.

What action then is the Department taking in this difficult area? To improve our knowledge of the needs of mentally disordered offenders, the Department of Health has commissioned research from Professor John Gunn into the treatment and security needs of patients in special hospitals and we look forward with keen anticipation to the results being available in 1991. This, together with his research into the mental health of the sentenced prisoner population,[1] will give us sound information on unmet need and on the appropriateness of the care some patients now receive.

As part of the mental illness initiative announced by Mr Freeman in July 1989, over the last few months we have been working, and we will continue to work, collaboratively with regional health authorities to identify the progress that has been made and the problems that have been encountered in implementing present policy. Our purpose is to identify what we at the centre need to do to help health authorities implement policy effectively. Particularly, we have been working with Mersey and South West Thames Regional Health Authorities to examine the possibility of collaborating on an assessment of unmet need.

The (Joint Home Office/Department of Health) Interdepartmental Working Group on Mentally Disturbed Offenders in the Prison System made a total of 16 wide-ranging recommendations, all of which have been accepted by the Government (Home Office, 1987b). The report really does provide a blueprint for future action and many of its proposals are being implemented. But we have a long way to go and both Departments are now focusing attention on the outstanding recommendations.

Unarguably more important even than service provision is prevention. What can be done to prevent illness and handicap, or to prevent mentally disordered people from offending. The general issue of prevention is one that we will be developing in months to come and time would not permit of my dealing with it in detail here. However, many mentally abnormal offenders are already known to the mental health service, often well-known over many years. The Spokes Report on the care and after-care of Sharon Campbell highlighted many of the difficulties in ensuring continuity of care for seriously mentally ill people when they leave hospital (DHSS, 1988). Anticipating the recommendations in Spokes, the Department of Health in its current planning guidelines requires all health authorities to establish by 31 March 1991 a 'care programme' approach to care outside hospital which will involve discharge planning, regular review, and the maintenance of some system to ensure that patients do not fall out of care into dereliction and crime (Department of Health, 1990).

Another aspect of prevention is the provision, for those who need it, of asylum; of a refuge from pressures that they cannot cope with. In planning this it is essential to realize that asylum can be found in many places other than large institutions. Here, particularly, it is vital to take account of the wishes of the disordered person. The unwillingness of mentally ill people who live on the streets to enter psychiatric hospitals even when their illness is severe enough to warrant admission is an indication of how severe a 'consumer resistance' problem can be.

At the present time, we have, in round numbers, 1700 beds in special hospitals, 500 beds in RSUs and 2000 beds in locked wards in mental illness and mental handicap hospitals, together with their supporting staff. However, we need to know whether these beds are appropriate in number and distributed most effectively.

Ministers are determined to provide a sensitive and flexible response to the widely differing needs of both mentally disordered offenders and other patients requiring treatment in secure conditions. The Department recognizes that now is the time to re-assess and evaluate all forms of secure provision and their relationships to one another and to psychiatric services generally. Although there is a paucity of currently available data, there is already evidence to suggest an overall shortfall in provision as well as inappropriate use and deployment of current facilities. A further pressing difficulty is obtaining timely and appropriate transfer from one facility to another whether between hospitals or from prison to hospital. Over the next two to three years the Department of Health will, with the help of colleagues in the Home Office and the wider forensic mental health world, be addressing these central issues. This task cannot be carried out in isolation and we will be looking for contributions from all those involved.

Discussion

Contributors discussed a number of themes concerning future provision for mentally disordered offenders; in particular, questions of research, resources and legislation.

Academic research and forensic psychiatry

It was suggested that, whilst forensic psychiatry had grown as a clinical specialty, there was little growth in associated academic research. Some current research projects were limited to relatively small samples. University input to research effort was necessary, but there was a problem in getting the Home Office, and the Departments of Health and of Education and Science to work together. There was a lack of co-ordination at central government level. The lack of available information and research resources was emphasized by another contributor. Although police forces were autonomous, there was a highly developed national research structure which could guide, but not direct them. Policing research was far in advance of that concerning mental health. The fact that there was little knowledge about numbers of mentally disordered offenders, was not acceptable. The difficulties in working across the boundaries between departments and divisions were emphasized.

Dr Reed acknowledged that the assessment of total populations was difficult, the work taking a number of years. It was not that information was suppressed, but that the knowledge was not available, partly because it was difficult satisfactorily to define mental disorder.

A more specific point was raised concerning the paucity of available information about practice on locked wards. There was an emphasis on the special hospitals and the regional secure units in research, but what was happening in the fields of general psychiatry and mental handicap? What was the history of these facilities? How much restraint was used, and were there effective substitutes? Did everyone in these facilities need to be locked up, and were suitable precautions taken to minimize their use?

Priorities of need and the co-ordination of services

It was observed that, although the Department of Health had a special interest in mental health, and special departments relating to it, this did not work through at the regional level, so the diversion of funds to other services was possible. Was a separate mental health service the answer? The White Paper (Department of Health, 1989*b*) might be relevant to this issue. Dr Reed responded that, with all its leaks, mental health remained in the right boat (with another contributor suggesting that it might however be a slow boat!). It was claimed that health authorities were facing great difficulties in setting priorities, with discovered needs out-stripping resources. Would the Department of Health force health authorities to establish these priorities? Dr Reed argued that it was for the health authorities to determine how they would use their resources, and that devolution of decision-making would continue. In response, it was claimed that devolution was an inadequate response to the needs of a marginalized group who required central direction and protection of services as a defence against pressures at the local level. The problem of targeting monies was acknowedged.

It was pointed out that the private sector had not become greatly involved in the long-term care of the mentally impaired. Where would this be provided in terms of the requirements set out in the Griffiths Report? (Griffiths, 1988). Would not a regional service be a better option than turning to the private sector? The private sector had proved to be adaptable and quick to respond to developing demands, but it was important not to overlook both the social and medical needs of the mentally impaired (Department of Health, 1989*c*).

It was suggested that there was no national co-ordination of services for mentally disordered offenders; they were peripheral to everyone's priorities. It was important to co-ordinate the views of the Department of Health with those of other professionals. Dr Reed argued that mentally disordered offenders were not a unique health group: their needs for care and containment were not essentially different from those of many others. In response, it was suggested that mentally disordered offenders might not have unique needs but they did face unique problems which arose out of their involvement in both the mental health and criminal justice systems. The problem posed by those who did not respond to treatment was addressed. Mental health services sometimes could not assist them; these services had to maintain the therapeutic endeavour, and the treatable within their care could not be combined with the non-treatable without the concept of care becoming corrupted. These 'non-copers' remained a group that no one knew how to help.

The impact of legislation

With current mental health legislation being primarily hospital-based, a question was raised about whether it was possible to develop legal provisions which extended control into community care and case management arrangements, and which would be broader than the specific proposal for community treatment orders.

It was suggested that it was necessary to look to the United States for evidence concerning community treatment orders. Some of the American systems might be unacceptable, but the condition of treatment as part of a probation order was an appropriate starting model, providing an element of compulsion in that failure to attend the doctor would result in the re-appraisal of the case. Another contributor emphasized that this arrangement would minimize the coercion involved in community treatment, and would thus allay the fears of some who resisted the idea. The possibility of the use of orders of guardianship was also floated. It was pointed out that provisions existed in Scotland for long-leave treatment orders. This could work for some moderately difficult individuals, but was of dubious benefit in the treatment of more difficult patients; it was impossible to treat someone in the community who was adamantly opposed to it. Another contributor pointed out that the problem with psychiatric treatment as a requirement of a probation order was that the consent of the patient was needed. In the case of chronic schizophrenics, this would require a long-term commitment to treatment which they might be unwilling to give.

Note
1. Now published in Gunn *et al.* (1991).

Part V
A concluding review

15

Future directions for research

W. WATSON

The papers and the subsequent discussions which made up the 1990
Cropwood Conference covered an enormous range of issues concerning
the situation of mentally disordered offenders in the era of community
care. It is not the purpose of these concluding remarks to summarize all
these issues, but to draw out certain important themes about which useful
comments might be made after the reflection induced by putting together
this report of proceedings. The whole conference effort remained true to
the brief of outlining possibilities for future provision. Indeed, the event
was remarkable for the tenacity and depth with which a broad, even
disparate group of committed people, all 'representatives of good practice', tackled the problems encountered in the provision of services for a
very marginalized client group. These comments will also be addressed
directly to issues central to the futures of this important minority of
disadvantaged citizens for whom both the psychiatric and criminal justice
systems must strive to cater.

Researching the current situation of mentally disordered offenders

Almost every participant demanded an increase in the quantity of
research undertaken concerning mentally disordered offenders. Indeed,
representatives of a number of bodies indicated their interest in sponsor-
ing or co-ordinating some of this effort. On what conceptual bases should
such work best be founded? Of course, a number of different methods
and perspectives will ideally be brought to bear on the issues. However,
one idea was referred to in many contexts; that of the mentally disordered
offender's 'career'. The concept renders inadequate any simple focus on
clearly delineated and significant episodes such as discharge from hospital, arrest, conviction, sentence, etc. There needs to be an attempt to

understand the complex ways in which some individuals become channelled through particular institutional and extra-institutional careers. When applied to the development of services, this approch can lead to a specific form of evaluation: how can future provision be organized, not merely so that it is flexible, and in some undefined way 'tailored' to the individual, but also so that the consequences of particular decisions do not create new forms of career structure which lead to or maintain the mentally disordered as an offender? Dr Fowles' paper, and the subsequent discussion, gave clear indication that routes to inappropriate placement cannot be deduced from a simple analysis of changes in global institutional statistics. The research effort needs to be put together 'on the ground', so as to reflect directly the experiences of mentally disordered offenders and the agencies with whom they make contact.

Within the sociological literature, there has been an attempt to displace the explanation for particular 'deviant' career structures away from the motivations and behaviours of the deviant subjects and into the patterns of interaction which characteristically obtain between the subject and his or her social and institutional environment. Indeed, such a perspective has informed both applied and more critical research on mentally disordered offenders (e.g. Menzies, 1987). The concept of career need not imply a reductive anti-psychiatry in which the internal psychological dynamics of the offender are marginalized in the process of explanation. Indeed, conventional psychiatric diagnoses and prognoses may prove to be important indicators of the likely direction of an individual's institutional career, regardless of whether he or she has been so 'labelled'.[1]

However, the ways in which particular types of career structure may become established necessarily involve contemporary changes in institutional and community provision for the mentally ill and the mentally handicapped, and this makes the task of formulating relevant research particularly difficult. In order to evaluate the impact of community care programmes on the situation of the mentally disordered who have offended in the past, or who are now offending, we cannot simply compare one set of careers (before decarceration) with another set (after decarceration), because many current careers involve the decarceration experience itself. The transcarceration hypothesis reduces the careers of putatively affected individuals either to a move from hospital to prison via the community or homelessness, or to a statistical shift in location from hospital to prison for the newly mentally disordered.

What is required is a detailed understanding of the life histories of people who may find themselves inappropriately embroiled with the criminal justice system for a variety of reasons, and after a variety of experiences. Needless to say, the processes by which some mentally disordered people become homeless need to be understood, but are by no means relevant to all mentally disordered offenders, and thus provide no explanation for the offending of many mentally disordered clients. The (often institutionalized) socially inadequate and rootless may form one population for whom the provision of community care is very difficult. However, providing community-based services for mentally disordered offenders, even those with established accommodation and work, is always problematic, given the difficulties in applying meaningful methods of control to those outside an institutional setting. The concept of career needs to be applied sensitively to individuals in a variety of situations, and not as a vehicle for a crude speculation that large numbers of people are being herded along one narrow track from the hospital to the prison. Research needs to proceed on the basis that mentally disordered offenders do not form an homogeneous group, sharing a unified sequence of experiences.

However, it may become apparent that certain common difficulties blight the lives of many. Perhaps more significant is the possibility that a number of groupings might be identified within the overall category, and where certain experiences or even definite career structures might be discerned. What would be the most likely axes around which such groupings might cluster? It may be highly probable that particular career trajectories would be associated with psychiatric diagnosis and type of offence, or a combination of the two. Of course, the careers of mentally handicapped offenders are likely to be quite unlike those of the mentally ill. However, it might also be the case that there are marked differences in the experiences of the sexes. There might also be important differences between those whose mental disorder or offending begins at an early age, and those for whom these events occur much later in life.

Indeed, a combination of these axes may provide the basis of forensic and nonspecialist psychiatric involvement with those accused and convicted of offences, with forensic specialists concentrating on patients with histories of acts or threats of serious violence, including a substantial minority diagnosed as suffering from a personality disorder. Other psychiatrists may become involved in the assessment and treatment of offenders associated with more minor offences, and whose characteristics might more closely match those of the general psychiatric in-patient and out-patient populations. Such a development would appear to constitute a useful division of labour. However, it would be important to investigate whether involvement with the forensic psychiatric services has a significant impact on the careers of patients (for better or worse), independent of any influence of variables of the above type.

It is through a sophisticated account of career patterns that the greatest understanding of the operation of race, sex and class biases might be established. Some notion of a disadvantaged career structure, rather than the experience of unconnected episodes of prejudicial treatment, might be invoked in explaining the over-representation of members of certain minority groups within the sentenced and restricted patient populations. Such an analysis need not shy away from identifying the locations where key decisions are taken which directly lead to structured disadvantages. However, tracing through differences in the situations of individuals arriving at these locations, and the variety of consequences which flow from such encounters could afford the most detailed understanding of overall patterns of representation.

The effects of diversion

The idea of diverting mentally disordered individuals away from the criminal justice system at the earliest stage of possible involvement (Home Office, 1990a) is based on an approach clearly related to that of an identifiable and mutable career structure. It was perhaps rather generally assumed in the foregoing papers and discussions that diversion from the criminal justice system would have a beneficial impact on the lives of most mentally disordered offenders.[2] If positive outcomes were always the case, the research efforts devoted to the evaluation of patient needs and those based on the attempt to understand patient's careers might be neatly dovetailed. 'Needs' would have to be viewed as a dynamic of possible requirements in the context of a predictable career, and in which clients' primary needs might be therapeutic and social direction away from particularly damaging paths. Conversely, the career could be defined, not just in terms of probable sequences of events, but also as an evolving pattern of individual needs. However, insofar as needs assessments are reliant upon patients' informed understanding of the social and therapeutic possibilities before them, the fullest assessment of the patients' needs would require their understanding of possibly unpalatable potential career structures.

Moreover, the impact of some types of involvement with criminal justice agencies might turn out to be associated with a more positive career structure than would be the case with diversion. Such a possibility would necessarily bring needs assessment into controversial territory, although this might be necessary for the needs of mentally disordered offenders to be fully evaluated. Practitioners and critics are aware that providing for mentally disordered offenders puts great strain on professional/client relationships, both because the welfare of others and of the public continually enter into the process of clinical judgement, and because the negotiation with the client over therapeutic provision is often conflictual, especially where medical professionals are effectively acting as agents of the courts. There is nothing in the development of an understanding of career structures among mentally disordered offenders which would necessarily serve to lessen these conflicts.

Thus, research into the careers of mentally disordered offenders will not diminish the practical and ethical problems which informed professionals already knowingly embrace, but it does provide an appropriate framework within which stringent evaluations of particular therapies, therapeutic placements, and social provisions can be generated. Furthermore, provisions for diversion might be critically examined, insofar as they might become integrated with known and yet to be established career patterns. This would be a important issue when dealing with those prone to violence. Typically, these evaluations are currently constructed through attenuated notion of career, with comparisons being made of rates of re-offending over a limited period of time, for example. These evaluations tell us very little about either the long-term, or the details of the real-life situations of those previously subject to particular therapeutic regimes, beyond whether or not they re-offend. Anecdotal evidence seems to suggest that many vulnerable individuals placed in 'the community' find themselves in quite unsupportive, even desperate, circumstances. It may be some time before the success or failure of therapeutic programmes designed to minimize the risk of offending behaviour can be ascertained. However, the processes by which these individuals can enter stressful personal circumstances are suitable objects of study in themselves, and may give some indication of future problems which, in turn, may help explain long-term processes of personal decline and eventual re-offending.

One method of provision which seems to be consistent with the career concept is that of case management. The close involvement of one professional with the overall circumstances of the client seems well designed to facilitate the perception and avoidance of sets of circumstances in which vulnerable people may become channelled along a damaging path. The evaluation of case management techniques would best be a comparison of career structures since the aim of case management is to 'bring together' the total welfare of the client over a period of time. Such evaluation therefore requires a comparison of careers within and without a case management structure, itself only possible with a coherent account of typical life-histories among mentally disordered offenders.

However, one note of caution needs to be sounded in advocating something like a case management approach. In so far as the case manager acts as advocate for the client, this is best achieved where he or she has funds to wield on the client's behalf. This may give the impression that if funds are 'shifted' to the case manager, facilities used by the client would compete for the capitations, thus ensuring the effective use of resources and the provision of effective therapies and services.

This is an over-simplification. First, facilities cannot be established through the provision of capitation, except where capitalization is provided on the basis of an expected income/profit from the provision of service. Thus, short of envisaging a situation where all provision is through the private sector, or through local and national authorities operating as a private sector, case management budgets are not going to provide the foundation of a system of funding. We heard at the conference how the private sector in the United Kingdom has typically responded to the existence of gaps in state provision which cause pressing problems for authorities in meeting their obligations. It seems certain that the backbone of comprehensive services for mentally disordered offenders will be maintained through the direct involvement of the state in setting up facilities which must be funded directly on the basis of the establishment of needs and the evaluation of their therapeutic programmes. The monies required for this are unlikely ever to come primarily from case management capitations, or the expectation of receiving them, although these capitations will come into the reckoning in establishing the direct revenue implications of running these services (for state, voluntary/charitable and private sectors). Thus, a far more complex pattern of funding is likely to develop with the emergence of case management approaches than might, at first, be apparent, and in which conventional local authority and national state capitalization remains significant.

Second, as has already been argued, the evaluation of services within a framework sensitive to the client's progress as a personal career requires a substantial and sophisticated research methodology. It seems unlikely that case managers would currently be in a position to make the judgments concerning available services, except on the basis of relatively crude indices of success and failure. Yet the case management system seems to be one remarkably compatible with the ideal of a far-sighted navigation of the client's life prospects. It would seem that case management would work best where services had been evaluated on the basis of their impact upon different types of clients' life histories. The leverage of holding individual budgets may work very well in ensuring that clients get the best service possible from care agencies, but does not, in itself, guarantee the promotion of more successful, and the demise or modification of less successful, services, an outcome which would typically require a research effort quite beyond the scope of individual case managers, but upon which they could hopefully draw. Indeed, such a developing body of research would form the informational content of both the interventions of case managers on behalf of individual clients, and the strategic decisions of overall service providers.

For a case management approach to be successful with mentally disordered offenders, it is essential that the courts become increasingly orientated to a career-based approach. This is, of course, already happening to a considerable degree, with the courts often being reluctant to initiate a course of action which might be detrimental to an offender in the long-term. The participation of courts in diversion schemes is explicit evidence of such an orientation. However, one problem needs to be addressed in promoting this development. Although an understanding of the impact of conviction upon a mentally disordered person might well involve the appreciation of the stigmatization that can follow from involvement with criminal justice agencies, the identification of an individual as being prone to a particular biographical trajectory might itself be highly stigmatizing. The courts may, at times, prefer to sentence the individual on the criteria of just deserts, taking mitigating psychiatric evidence into account, rather than to mark the person down as a problem in the long-term. The involvement of criminal justice and care agencies in the lives of mentally disordered offenders seems to require a sophisticated resolve to confront the potentially disastrous consequencies of what might appear straightforward and limited punitive decisions, while at the same time remaining aware that this knowledge can not make resultant decisions innocent of the potential to have negative consequences for mentally disordered people found guilty of criminal offences.

The ethics of intervention in the era of community care

The foregoing discussion raises, but leaves unanswered, a series of questions concerning the jurisprudence of the mentally disordered offender. It has already been suggested that the courts do not adhere to a deductively 'principled' approach in which justice is seen as inherent in the legal response to offences as such, even when mitigating circumstances are taken into account. What we see is a complex, practical jurisprudence in which the basic criterion is a morality of predictable consequences. For these purposes, the courts need clear evidence concerning the effectiveness of treatments provided for mentally disordered offenders, particularly where a diminution of the risk of violence or self-injury is an explicit aim of the treatment and an expectation of the court. All those involved in the care of mentally disordered offenders, especially when the offences involve violence, remain aware that treatment cannot always be the only aim of provision. Some will hold that punishment remains a legitimate objective for some mentally disordered individuals, not simply as a kind of 'treatment', but as an act of retribution. In any case, there are clearly circumstances in which the containment of risk must be given a high priority. In these situations the necessity for a sound evaluation of the efficacy of treatment programmes is not marginalized, but is paramount, and it is within the context of the whole career of the mentally disordered offender that effective treatment becomes synonymous with the containment of risk.

The relation between the hospital, the prison and the community remained at the centre of many of the foregoing discussions. Where the aim of a decarceration programme is seen as providing opportunity for the patient to experience a proper 'life', rather than merely to shift the location of care, the prison can legitimately be seen as a part of the normal (extra-hospital) community. The individual acquires decision-making opportunities which necessarily imply responsibility, and detention within the penal system can be the result of conduct for which such a person has become responsible. At the same time, there was general agreement at the conference that the hospital can become part of the community where organizational barriers between the possibilities of independent existence in the community and the asylum provided within an institutional setting can be dismantled. Clearly, a case manager might be in a position to negotiate rapid admission to a place of asylum for a vulnerable client.

However, one serious problem which was raised on a number of occasions concerned the practical and ethical difficulties in establishing systems which allow both psychiatric health care and criminal justice practitioners to intervene more directly in the lives of mentally disordered offenders without the disaster of imprisonment or an unnecessary confinement in hospital. How practical and acceptable are arrangements in which health care professionals or probation officers effectively contain and supervise individuals within a community setting? A number of relatively discrete moral questions might be raised here, such as the impact on the human dignity of a person subject to rather public systems of supervision, for example the requirement to reside in a specialist hostel, or the disclosure of information to employers. However, the focus of these concluding remarks will be on the relation of the morality of any systems of community containment to the concept of the career.

Every moral judgment which must be made concerning the treatment of, and social provision for, the mentally disordered offender is necessarily a balance of competing imperatives; the fundamental condition of entry into the arena of effective involvement with this marginalized group. Certain legal guarantees must remain which inhere in the individual's status as a citizen. There can be no diminution of this status if new systems appropriate to the outreach of forensic psychiatry services into the community are to be acceptable. However, systems cannot be morally evaluated in these terms alone. Evaluation of the effectiveness of any new legal provision and related system of care is integral to an account of the acceptability of particular arrangements. These issues can only be confronted through an understanding of the influence of different arrangements on the careers of those subject to their provisions. The parts played by hospitalization, arrest and imprisonment in the lives of some of our society's most vulnerable members are yet to be fully understood. Any new medico-legal arrangements consistent with the ethos of community living cannot be evaluated simply on the basis that new liberties must be beneficial, or that new constraints must be pernicious. The stigmas of both indictment for offence and of psychiatric diagnosis are the lot of the individuals whose care has been so fully discussed at this conference. Any new system envisaged for their care and containment within the community cannot be evaluated fully without a detailed understanding of the impact of these services over the long-term for the offenders formally required to participate in them. The degree to which such systems are successful in managing the stigmas from which their clients inevitably suffer cannot simply be a matter of claiming that freedom outside hospital or prison must be better than a period within an institution, or even that public containment must be more humiliating than segregation. Detailed research on the complex impact of the new systems must form the basis of any such judgment. The future developments in provision envisaged in the Government's major review of services, predicted at the end of Dr Reed's paper, and now completed by the Department of Health and Home Office (1991), will require this research and critical analysis.

Notes
1. Research identifying the mentally ill among prison populations may indicate that this is so, although many have had a previous involvement with psychiatric services (see the chapter by Dr Fowles in this volume).
2. Although there was recognition of the possible negative consequences of a psychiatric diagnosis for those formally detained within institutions under sections of the Mental Health Act 1983 (see especially the chapter by Dr Peay in this volume).

References

Adler, F. (1986). Jail as a repository for former mental patients. *International Journal of Offender Therapy and Comparative Criminology, 30*, 225–36.

Ahmed, S., Cheetham, J. & Small, J. (eds.) (1986). *Social Work with Black Children and their Families*. London: Batsford (in association with British Agencies for Adopting and Fostering).

American Friends Service Committee (1971). *Struggle for Justice*. New York: Hill and Wang.

Anthony, W. A., Cohen, M., Farkas, M. & Cohen, B. F. (1988). Case management – more than a response to a dysfunctional system. *Community Mental Health Journal, 24*, 219–28.

Audit Commission (1986). *Making a Reality of Community Care*. London: HMSO.

Bachrach, L. L. & Lamb, H. R. (1989). What have we learned from de-institutionalization? *Psychiatric Annals, 19*, 12–21.

Bagley, C. (1976). Behavioural deviance in ethnic minority children. *New Community, 5*, 230.

Bean, P. (1986). *Mental Disorder and Legal Control*. Cambridge: Cambridge University Press.

Bean, P. & Mounser, L. (1989). Community care and the discharge of patients from mental hospitals. *Law, Medicine and Health Care, 17*, 166–73.

Bebbington, P. E., Hurry, J. & Tennant, C. (1981). Psychiatric disorders in selected immigrant groups in Camberwell. *Social Psychiatry, 16*, 43–51.

Binns, J. K., Carlisle, J. M., Nimmo, D. H., Park, R. & Todd, N. A. (1969). Remanded in custody for psychiatric examination: a review of 83 cases and a comparison with those remanded in hospital. *British Journal of Psychiatry, 115*, 1133–9.

Bluglass, R. (1978). Regional secure units and interim security for psychiatric patients. *British Medical Journal, 1*, 489–93.

Bluglass, R. (1985). The recent Mental Health Act in the United Kingdom: issues and perspectives. In Roth, M. & Bluglass, R. (eds.) *Psychiatry, Human Rights and the Law*, 21–31. Cambridge: Cambridge University Press.

Bond, G.R., Miller, L. D., Krumwied, R. D., & Ward, R. S. (1988). Assertive case management in three CMHCs: a controlled study. *Hospital and Community Psychiatry, 39*, 411–18.

Boothroyd, J. (1988). The prisoners we are failing. *Police Review*, 8 July, 1426–7.

Bottoms, A. E. & McWilliams, W. (1979). A non-treatment paradigm for probation practice. *British Journal of Social Work*, **9**, 159–202.

Bowden, P. (1978). Men remanded into custody for medical reports: the selection for treatment. *British Journal of Psychiatry*, **132**, 320–31.

Bowden, P. (1983). Madness or badness. *British Journal of Hospital Medicine*, **30**, 388–94.

Brahams, D. & Weller, M. (1985a). Crime and homelessness among the mentally ill – I. *New Law Journal*, 28 June, 626–7.

Brahams, D. & Weller, M. (1985b). Crime and homelessness among the mentally ill – II. *New Law Journal*, 26 July, 761–3.

Brewin, C. R. & Wing, J. K. (1988). *The MRC Needs for Care Assessment Manual*. Second edition. London: Institute of Psychiatry – MRC Social Psychiatry Unit.

Brewin, C. R., Wing, J. K., Mangen, S., Brugha, T. S. & MacCarthy, B. (1987). Principles and practice of measuring needs in the long-term mentally ill: the MRC needs for care assessment. *Psychological Medicine*, **17**, 971–81. London: Institute of Psychiatry – MRC Social Psychiatry Unit.

Brooks, A. D. (1984). Defining the dangerousness of mentally ill: involuntary civil commitment. In Craft, M. & Craft, A. (eds.) *Mentally Abnormal Offenders*, 280–307. London: Ballière Tindall.

Brown, D. (1989). *Detention at the Police Station under the Police and Criminal Evidence Act 1984*. London: HMSO.

Brown, G. W., Bone, M., Dalison, B. & Wing, J. K. (1966). *Schizophrenia and Social Care*. London: Oxford University Press.

Brugha, T. S., Wing, J. K., Brewin, C. R., MacCarthy, B., Mangen, S. P., Lesage, A. & Munford, J. (1988). The problems of people in long-term psychiatric day care. *Psychological Medicine*, **18**, 443–56.

Burke, A. (1984). Racism and psychological disturbance among West Indians in Britain. *International Journal of Social Psychiatry*, **30**, 50–68.

Burt, C. (1925). *The Young Delinquent*. London: University of London Press.

Cavadino, M. (1989). *Mental Health Law in Context: doctors' orders*. Aldershot: Dartmouth.

Chiswick, D. (1985). Use and abuse of psychiatric testimony. *British Medical Journal*, **290**, 975–7.

Clare, A. W. (1980). *Psychiatry in Dissent: controversial issues in thought and practice*. Second edition. London: Tavistock.

Coard, B. (1977). *How the West Indian Child is made Eductionally Subnormal in the British School System*. London: New Beacon Books.

Cochrane, R. (1971). Mental illness in immigrants to England and Wales: an analysis of mental hospital admissions. *Social Psychiatry*, **12**, 25–35.

Coid, J. (1987). Criminalizing the Mentally Ill. Dissertation for the Diploma in Criminology. London: University of London.

Coid, J. (1988a). Mentally abnormal prisoners on remand: I – rejected or accepted by the NHS? *British Medical Journal*, **296**, 1779–82.

Coid, J. (1988b). Mentally abnormal prisoners on remand: II – comparison of services provided by Oxford and Wessex Regions. *British Medical Journal*, **296**, 1783–4.

Connah, B. & Lancaster, S. (1989). *The NHS Handbook*. London: MacMillan Press Ltd.

Creer, C. & Wing, J. K. (1974). *Schizophrenia at Home*. Surbiton: National Schizophrenia Fellowship.

Croft J. (1978). *Research in Criminal Justice*: Home Office research study No 44. London: HMSO.

Dell, S. (1983). Wanted: an insanity defence that can be used. *Criminal Law Review*, 431–7.

Dell, S. & Gibbens T. C. N. (1971). Remand of women offenders for medical reports. *Medicine, Science and the Law*, **11**, 117–27.

Dell, S. and Robertson, G. (1988). *Sentenced to Hospital: offenders in Broadmoor*. Maudsley Monograph No 32. London: Oxford University Press.

Department of Health (1989a). *Caring for People: community care in the next decade and beyond* (Cm 849). London: HMSO.

Department of Health (1989b). *Working for Patients* (Cm 555). London: HMSO.

Department of Health (1989c). *Needs and Responses: services for adults with mental handicap who are mentally ill, who have behaviour problems or who offend*. London: Department of Health.

Department of Health (1990). *The Care Programme Approach for People with a Mental Illness Referred to the Specialist Psychiatric Services*. Circular HC (90)23. London: Department of Health.

Department of Health/Home Office (1991). *Review of Health and Social Services for Mentally Disordered Offenders and Others Requiring Similar Services. The Reports of the Service Advisory Groups: an overview with glossary*. London: Department of Health.

Department of Health and Welsh Office (1990). *Code of Practice: Mental Health Act 1983*. London: HMSO.

Department of Health and Social Security (1971a). *Hospital Services for the Mentally Ill*. Hospital Memorandum No 97. London: DHSS.

Department of Health and Social Security (1971b). *Better Services for the Mentally Handicapped*. London: HMSO.

Department of Health and Social Security (1974a). *Security in NHS Hospitals for the Mentally Ill and the Mentally Handicapped*. Health Service Circular No 87. London: DHSS.

Department of Health and Social Security (1974b). *Interim Report of the Committee on Mentally Abnormal Offenders* (Cm 5698). London: HMSO.

Department of Health and Social Security (1974c). *Revised Report of the Working Party on Security in NHS Psychiatric Hospitals*. London: DHSS.

Department of Health and Social Security (1975). *Better Services for the Mentally Ill*. London: HMSO.

Department of Health and Social Security (1988). *Report of the Committee of Enquiry into the Care and Aftercare of Miss Sharon Campbell* (Cm 440). London: HMSO.

Department of Health and Social Security, Home Office, Welsh Office and Lord Chancellor's Department (1978). *Review of the Mental Health Act 1959* (Cm 7320). London: HMSO.

Dickens, B. M. (1985). Prediction, professionalism and public policy. In Webster, C., Ben-Aron, M. & Hucker, S. (eds.) *Dangerousness: Probability and Prediction, Psychiatry and Public Policy*. Cambridge: Cambridge University Press.

Donzelot, J. (1979). *The Policing of Families*. London: Hutchinson.

Edwards, G., Williamson, V., Hawker, A., Hensman, C. & Postoyan, S. (1986). Census of a reception centre. *British Journal of Psychiatry*, **114**, 1031–9.

Emerson, E., Toogood, A., Monsell, J., Barrett, S., Bell, C., Cummings, R. & McCool, C. (1987). Challenging behaviour and community services: I – introduction and overview. *Mental Handicap*, **15**, 166–8.

Faulk, M. and Trafford, P. (1975). Efficacy of medical remands. *Medicine, Science and the Law*, **15**, 276–9.

Fennell, P. (1992). Community treatment orders and patient safeguards: trends and transformations in mental health law. *International Journal of Law and Psychiatry*, **15**. (In press.)

Fisher, G., Landis, D. & Clark, K. (1988). Case management, service provision and client change. *Community Mental Health Journal*, **24**, 134–42.

Genders, E. & Player, E. (1989). *A Study of the Therapeutic Regime at Grendon Prison*. Report for the Home Office. Oxford: Oxford Centre for Criminological Research.

Gibbens, T. C. N., Soothill, K. & Pope, P. (1977). *Medical Remands in the Criminal Court*, Maudsley Monograph No 25. London: Oxford Univerity Press.

Goering, P. N., Wasylenki, D. A., Farkas, M., Lancee, W. J. & Ballantyne, R. (1988). What difference does case management make? *Hospital and Community Psychiatry*, **39**, 272–82.

Goffman, E. (1961). *Asylums: essays on the social situation of mental patients and other inmates*. New York: Anchor Books.

Gostin, L. (1983). Contemporary legal approaches to psychiatry in mental disorder and the law: effects of the new legislation. In Shapland, J. & Williams, T. (eds.) *Issues in Criminological and Legal Psychology*, No 4. Leicester: British Psychological Society.

Griew, E. (1984). Let's implement Butler on mental disorder and crime! *Current Legal Problems*, **31**, 47–58.

Griffiths, R. (1988). *Community Care – Agenda for Action*. London: HMSO.

Grounds, A. T. (1987). The detention of 'psychopathic disorder' patients in special hospitals: critical issues. *British Journal of Psychiatry*, **151**, 474–8.

Gudeman, J. E. & Shore, M. F. (1984). Beyond de-institutionalization: a new class of facilities for the mentally ill. *New England Journal of Medicine*, **311**, 832–6.

Gunn, J., Robertson, G., Dell, S. & Way, C. (1978). *Psychiatric Aspects of Imprisonment*. London: Academic Press.

Gunn, J. & Taylor, P. J. (1983). Rehabilitation of the mentally abnormal offender. In Watts, F. N. & Bennett, D. H. (eds.) *Theory and Practice of Psychiatric Rehabilitation*, 115–128. Chichester: Wiley.

Gunn, J., Maden, A. & Swinton, M. (1991). *Mentally Disordered Prisoners*. London: Home Office.

Hajioff, J. (1989). Managing mentally abnormal offenders. *Psychiatric Bulletin of the Royal College of Psychiatrists*, **13**, 480–1.

Hale, N. (1989). *Social Inquiry Reports at Horseferry Road Magistrates' Court* (a project by the Community Resources Team at Borough High Street). London: Inner London Probation Service.

Harris, M. & Bergman, H. C. (1987). Case management with the chronically mentally ill: a clinical perspective. *American Journal of Orthopsychiatry*, **57**, 296–302.

Harrison, G., Owens, D., Holton, A. & Neilson, D. (1988). A prospective study of severe mental disorder in Afro-Caribbean patients. *Psychological Medicine*, **18**, 643–57.

Herridge, C. (1989). Treatment of psychotic patients in prison. *Psychiatric Bulletin of the Royal College of Psychiatrists,* **13**, 200–1.

Higgins, J. (1988). *The Business of Medicine: private health care in Britain.* Basingstoke: MacMillan Education.

Hill, D. (1969). *Psychiatry in Medicine.* London: Nuffield Provincial Hospitals Trust.

Hirsch, S. R. (1988). *Psychiatric Beds and Resources: factors influencing bed use and service planning.* Report to the Royal College of Psychiatrists. London: Gaskell.

Hitch, P. J. & Clegg, P. (1980). Modes of referral of overseas immigrant and native born first admissions to psychiatric hospital. *Social Science and Medicine,* **14**, 369–74.

HMSO (1969). *Report of the Committee of Inquiry into allegations of ill-treatment of patients and other irregularities at the Ely Hospital, Cardiff* (Cm 3975). London: HMSO.

HMSO (1972). *Report of the Committee of Inquiry into Whittingham Hospital* (Cm 4861). London: HMSO.

Hollin, C. (1989). *Psychology and Crime: an introduction to criminological psychology.* London: Routledge.

Home Office (1926). *Royal Commission on Lunacy and Mental Disorder* (Cm 2700). London: HMSO.

Home Office (1978). *Research in Criminal Justice.* Home Office Research Study No 44. London: HMSO.

Home Office (1978). *Survey of the South East Prison Population.* Home Office Research Bulletin No 5. London: HMSO.

Home Office (1979). *Hostels for Offenders.* Home Office Research Study No 52. London: HMSO.

Home Office (1985). *Report of the Committee on the Prison Disciplinary System.* London: HMSO.

Home Office (1986a). *Offenders Suffering from Psychopathic Disorder.* London: HMSO.

Home Office (1986b). *The Prison Disciplinary System in England and Wales* (Cm 9920). London: HMSO.

Home Office (1987a). *Criminal Statistics, England and Wales Supplementary Tables,* Vol 5. London: Government Statistical Service.

Home Office (1987b). *Report of the Interdepartmental Working Group of Home Office and DHSS Officials on Mentally Disturbed Offenders in the Prison System in England and Wales.* London: HMSO.

Home Office (1988a). *Private Sector Involvement in the Remand System.* London: HMSO.

Home Office (1988b). *Punishment, Custody and the Community* (Cm 424). London: HMSO.

Home Office (1988c). *Prison Statistics England and Wales 1987* (Cm 547). London: HMSO.

Home Office (1988d). *The Parole System in England and Wales: Report of the Review Committee* (Cm 532). London: HMSO.

Home Office (1989a). *Report on the Work of the Prison Service April 1988-March 1989.* London: HMSO.

Home Office (1989b). *Bail Accommodation and Secure Bail Hostels, a consultative paper.* London: Home Office.

Home Office (1990*a*). *Provision for Mentally Disordered Offenders*, Circular 66/90. London: Home Office.

Home Office (1990*b*). *Scrutiny Report on the Prison Medical Service*. London: Home Office.

Home Office (1991). *Prison Disturbances April 1990. Report of an Inquiry* (Cm 1456). London: HMSO.

Home Office/Department of Health and Social Security (1975). *Report to the Committee on Mentally Disordered Offenders* (Cm 6244). London: HMSO.

Hoult, J. (1986). Community care of the acutely mentally ill. *British Journal of Psychiatry*, **149**, 137–44.

House of Commons (1985). *Second Paper from the Social Services Select Committee Session 1984–1985. Community Care with Special Reference to Adult Mentally Ill and Mentally Handicapped People*. London: HMSO.

House of Commons Social Services Committee (1986). *Session 1985–86 Prison Medical Service* (HC 72-I). London: HMSO.

Inner London Education Authority (1981). *Ethnic Census of School Support Centres and Educational Guidance Centres* (RS/784/81). London: ILEA.

Inner London Education Authority (1985). *Schools Support Programme: the re-integration of pupils into mainstream schools* (RS/068/85). London: ILEA.

Intagliata, J. (1982). Improving the quality of community care for the chronically mentally disabled: the role of case management. *Schizophrenia Bulletin*, **8**, 655–74.

Jarman, B. (1983). Identification of underprivileged areas. *British Medical Journal*, **286**: 1705–9.

Jarman, B. (1984). Underprivileged areas: validation and distribution of scores. *British Medical Journal*, **289**, 1587–92.

Johnstone, E. C., Owens, D. G. C., Gold, A., Crow, T. J. & MacMillan, J. F. (1984). Schizophrenia patients discharged from hospital – a follow-up study. *British Journal of Psychiatry*, **145**, 586–90.

Jones, T. (1989). What they left out. *Health Service Journal*, **99**, 1368–9.

Jones, T. & Young, J. (1989). Why aren't the police out catching burglars? *The Guardian*, 28 August.

Kilgour, J. C. (1984). The prison medical service in England and Wales. *British Medical Journal*, **288**, 1603–5.

King, M. (1981). *The Framework of Criminal Justice*. London: Croom Helm.

King, R. and Morgan, R. (1980). *The Future of the Prison System*. London: Gower.

Kneesworth House Hospital (1989). *Kneesworth House Hospital* Clinical Brochure. Bassingbourn-cum-Kneesworth, Royston, Hertfordshire.

Konecni, V., Milcahy, E. & Ebbesen, E. (1980). Prison or hospital: factors affecting the processing of persons suspected of being 'mentally disordered sex offenders'. In Sales, B. & Lipsitt, P. (eds.) *New Directions in Psychological Research*, 87–124. New York: Van Nostrand Reinhold.

Kramer, M. (1989). The biostatistical approach. In Williams, P., Wilkinson, G. & Rawnsley, K. (eds.) *The Scope of Epidemiological Psychiatry*, 86–107. London: Routledge.

Laing & Buisson Publications (1987). *Laing's Review of Private Healthcare 1987*. London: Laing and Buisson.

Law Commission (1989). *A Criminal Code for England and Wales* (Law Com No 143). London: HMSO.

Leach, J. & Wing, J. K. (1980). *Helping Destitute Men*. London: Tavistock.

Leff, J. (1986). Planning a community psychiatric service: from theory to practice. In Wilkinson, G. & Freeman, H. (eds.) *The Provision of Mental Health Services in Britian: the way ahead*. London: Gaskell.

Littlewood, R. (1981). *Aliens and Alienists – ethnic minorities and psychiatry*. Harmondsworth: Penguin.

Littlewood, R. & Lipsedge, M. (1981). Acute psychotic reactions in Caribbean-born patients. *Psychological Medicine*, **11**, 303–18.

Longman Group (1988). *The Directory of Independent Hospitals and Health Services*. London: Longman Group UK Ltd.

Mason, P. (1984). Services for the mentally abnormal offender: an overview. In Shapland, J. & Williams, T. (eds.) *Issues in Criminological and Legal Psychology*, No 6, 12–16. Leicester: British Psychological Society.

Matthew, G. K. (1971). Measuring need and evaluating services. In McLachlan, G. (ed.) *Portfolio for Health: problems and progress in medical care*. Sixth series. London: Oxford University Press.

Maxwell, A. E. (1970). *Basic Statistics in Behavioural Reseach*. Harmondsworth: Penguin.

McBarnet, D. (1981). *Conviction: Law, the State and the Construction of Justice*. London: Macmillan.

McKittrick, N. (1987). Prison discipline – Government steps back. *Justice of the Peace*, **151**, 739–40.

Mental Health Act Commission (1989). *Third Biennial Report 1987–89*. London: HMSO.

Menzies, R. (1987). The dynamics of psychiatric discretion: order and disorder in a pre-trial forensic clinic. Paper presented at the 1987 Annual Meeting of the American Society of Criminology, Montreal, Quebec.

Meuller, J. & Hopp, M. (1987). Attitudinal, administrative, legal and fiscal barriers to case management in social rehabilitation of the mentally ill. *International Journal of Mental Health*, **15**, 44–58.

National Association for the Care and Resettlement of Offenders (1985). *Black People in the Criminal Justice System*. NACRO Briefing Paper March 1985. London: NACRO.

NHS Hospital Advisory Service/Social Services Inspectorate (1988). *Report on Services provided by Broadmoor Hospital*. London: Department of Health.

National Unit for Psychiatric Research and Development (1989). *Evaluating the closure of Cane Hill Hospital: plans for residential services and the long-stay population: interim report*. Mimeo. London: NUPRD.

Owens, P. and Glennerster, H. (1990). *Nursing in Conflict*. London: Macmillan Education.

Packer, H. (1969). *The Limits of the Criminal Sanction*. Stanford: Stanford University Press.

Parker, E. (1980). Mentally disordered offenders and their protection from punitive sanctions: the English experience. *International Journal of Law and Psychiatry*, **3**, 461–70.

Peay, J. (1988). Offenders suffering from psychopathic disorder: the rise and demise of a consultation document. *British Journal of Criminology*, **28**, 67–81.

Peay, J. (1989). *Tribunals on Trial: a study of decision-making under the Mental Health Act 1983*. Oxford: Clarendon Press.

Penrose, L. S. (1939). Mental disease and crime: outline of a study of European statistics. *British Journal of Medical Psychology*, **18**, 1–15.

Penrose, L. S. (1943). A note on the statistical relationship between mental deficiency and crime in the United States. *American Journal of Mental Deficiency*, **47**, 462–6.

Pollitt, C. (1989). Consuming Passions. *Health Service Journal*, **99**, 1436–7.

Potas (1982). *Just Deserts for the Mad*. Canberra: Australian Institute of Criminology.

Prins, H. (1980). *Offenders, Deviants or Patients?* London: Tavistock.

Prins, H. (1982). *Criminal Behaviour*. London: Tavistock.

Prins, H. (1988). Dangerous clients: further observations on the limitation of mayhem. *British Journal of Social Work*, **18**, 593–609.

Prins, H. (1990). Mental abnormality and criminality – an uncertain relationship. *Medicine, Science and the Law*, **30**, 247–58.

Prins, H. (1991). *Bizarre Behaviours: boundaries of psychiatric disorder*. London: Tavistock/Routledge.

Richardson, G. (1988). Prisoners, patients and the right to fair process. Paper presented to the British Society of Criminology, London, 21 September 1988.

Robertson, G. (1982). The 1959 Mental Health Act of England and Wales: changes in the use of its criminal provisions. In Gunn, J. & Farrington, D. (eds.) *Abnormal Offenders, Delinquency, and the Criminal Justice System*, Vol 1, 245–268. Chichester: Wiley.

Rogers, A. and Faulkner, A. (1987). *A Place of Safety*. London: MIND.

Rollin, H. (1969). *The Mentally Abnormal Offender and the Law*. London: Pergamon.

Roth, M. (1985). The historical background: the past 25 years since the Mental Health Act 1959. In Roth, M. & Bluglass, R. (eds.) *Psychiatry, Human Rights and The Law*, 1–8. Cambridge: Cambridge University Press.

Royal College of Psychiatrists (1980). *Secure Facilities for Psychiatric Patients: a comprehensive policy*. London: Royal College of Psychiatrists.

Rwegellera, G. G. C. (1977). Psychiatric morbidity among West Africans and West Indians living in London. *Psychological Medicine*, **7**, 317–29.

Scannell, T. D. (1989). Community care and the difficult and offender patient. *British Journal of Psychiatry*, **154**, 615–19.

Scott, P. D. (1967). *Royal Commission on the Penal System in England and Wales: written evidence of the Institute of Psychiatry*, Vol 2, 147–8. London: HMSO.

Scott, P. D. (1974). Solutions to the problem of the dangerous offender. *British Medical Journal*, **4**, 640–1.

Scull, A. T. (1989). *Social Order/Mental Disorder: Anglo-American psychiatry in historical perspective*. London: Routledge.

Shapland, S. and Williams, T. (1983). The scope of the new legislation. In Shapland, J. & Williams, T. (eds.) *Issues in Criminological and Legal Psychology*, No 4, 6–14. Leicester: British Psychological Society.

Sims, A. C. P. and Symonds, R. L. (1975). Psychiatric referrals from the police. *British Journal of Psychiatry*, **127**, 171–81.

Steadman, H. J., Monahan, J., Duffee, B., Hartstone, E. & Robbins, P. C. (1984). The impact of state hospital de-institutionalization on United States prison populations, 1968–78. *Journal of Criminal Law and Criminology*, **75**, 474–90.

Steadman, H. J. & Morrissey, J. P. (1987). The impact of de-institutionalization on the criminal justice system: implications for understanding changing modes of social control. In Lowman, J., Menzies, R. J. & Palys, T. S. (eds). *Transcarceration: essays in the sociology of social control*, 227–249. Aldershot: Gower.

Stein, L. I. & Test, M. A. (1985). *The Training in Community Living Model: a decade of experience*. San Francisco: Jossey Bass.

Stephen, M. (1988). Problems of police/social work interaction: some American lessons. *Howard Journal of Criminal Justice*, **27**, 81–91.

Stone, C. E. (1988). *Bail Information for the Crown Prosecution Service*. Final report on the Probation Initiative 'Diversion from Custody and Prosecution' Vol 1. New York: Vera Institute of Justice.

Stone, C. E. (1989). *Public Interest Case Assessment*. Report on the Probation Initiative 'Diversion from Custody and Prosecution', Vol 2. New York: Vera Institute of Justice.

Taylor, P. (1985). Motives for offending among violent and psychotic men. *British Journal of Psychiatry*, **147**, 491–8.

Taylor, P, J. (1986). Psychiatric disorders in London's life sentenced offenders. *British Journal of Criminology*, **26**, 63–78.

Taylor, P. J. & Gunn, J. (1984*a*). Violence and psychosis – risk of violence among psychotic men. *British Medical Journal*, **288**, 1945–9.

Taylor, P. J. & Gunn, J. (1984*b*). Violence and psychosis – effect of psychiatric diagnosis on conviction and sentencing of offenders. *British Medical Journal*, **289**, 9–12.

Teplin, L. A. & Pruett, N. S. (1992). Police as street corner psychiatrists: managing the mentally ill. *International Journal of Law and Psychiatry*, **15** 139–56.

Test, M. A. (1979). Continuity of care. In Stein, L. I. (ed.) *Community Support Systems for the Long-Term Patient*. San Francisco: Jossey Bass.

Thornicroft, G. & Bebbington, P. (1989). De-institutionalization – from hospital closure to service development. *British Journal of Psychiatry*, **155**, 739–53.

Tidmarsh, D. & Wood, S. (1972). Psychiatric aspects of destitution: a study of the Camberwell Reception Centre. In Wing, J. K. & Hailey, A. M. (eds.) *Evaluating a Community Psychiatic Service. The Camberwell Register 1964–1971*, 327–342. London: Oxford University Press.

Tooth, G. C. & Brooke, E. M. (1961). Trends in the mental hospital population and their effect on future planning. *Lancet*, **i**, 710.

Turner, T. (1988). Community care. *The British Journal of Psychiatry*, **152**, 1–3.

UK Government (1987). *Reply to the Third Report from the Social Services Committee Session 1985/86* (Cm 115). London: HMSO.

Vagg, J. (1987). *Support for Difficult to Place People in Oxford: proposals for action*. Oxford: The Elmore Committee.

Verdun-Jones, S. (1989). Sentencing the partly mad and the partly bad: the case of the hospital order in England and Wales. *International Journal of Law and Psychiatry*, **12**, 1–27.

Wade, H. (1988). *Administrative Law*. London: Oxford University Press.

Walker, N. D. (1977). *Behaviour and Misbehaviour: explanations and non-explanations*. Oxford: Blackwells.

Walker, N. & McCabe, S. (1973). *Crime and Insanity in England*, Vol 2. Edinburgh: Edinburgh University Press.

Washbrook, R. A. H. (1981). Neuroticism and offenders. *International Journal of Offender Therapy and Comparative Criminology,* **24**, 122–9.

Watson, S. (1986). Changes in the use of psychiatric reports in magistrates' Courts. Unpublished MPhil Thesis, University of York.

Weller, M. P. I. (1989). Mental illness – who cares? *Nature,* **339**, 248–52.

Weller, M. P. I. & Weller, B. G. A. (1988). Crime and mental illness. *Medicine, Science and the Law,* **28**, 38–46.

Whitehouse, P. (1983). Race, bias and social enquiry reports. *Probation Journal,* **30**, 43–9.

Windlesham Lord (1989). Life sentences: the paradox of indeterminacy. *Criminal Law Review*, 244–256.

Wing, J. K. (ed.) (1982). Long-term community care: experience in a London borough. *Psychological Medicine*, Monograph Supplement, No 2. Cambridge: Cambridge University Press.

Wing, J. K. (ed.) (1989*a*). *Health Services Planning and Research.* London: Gaskell.

Wing, J. K. (1989*b*). The measurement of social disablement. The MRC Social Behaviour and Social Role Performance Schedules. *Social Psychiatry and Epidemiology,* **24**, 173–8.

Wing, J. K. (1990*a*). Community care: vision and reality. Paper presented at the proceedings of the Malvern Conference on the closure of Powick.

Wing, J. K. (1990*b*). Meeting the needs of people with psychiatric disorders. *Social Psychiatry and Psychiatric Epidemiology,* **25**, 2–8.

Wing, J. K. & Bennett, C. (1989). *Long-Term Care in the Worcester Development Project. Report on Research.* Report to the Department of Health and Social Security.

Wing, J. K. & Brown, G. W. (1970). *Institutionalism and Schizophrenia.* London: Cambridge University Press.

Wing, J. K. & Hailey, A. M. (eds.) (1972). *Evaluating a Community Psychiatric Service. The Camberwell Register, 1964–1971.* London: Oxford University Press.

Wing, J. K. & Olsen, R. (eds.) (1979). *Community Care for the Mentally Disabled.* London: Oxford University Press.

Wing, L. (1989). *Hospital Closure and the Resettlement of Residents.* London: Avebury/Gower.

Women's Equality Group/London Strategic Policy Unit (Greater London Council) (1985). *Breaking the Silence: women's imprisonment.* London: LSPU.

Wood Sir J. (1985). Detention of patients: administrative problems facing mental health review tribunals. In Roth, M. & Bluglass, R. (eds.) *Psychiatry, Human Rights and the Law*, 114–122. Cambridge: Cambridge University Press.

Wykes, T. (1982). A hostel ward for 'new' long-stay patients: an evaluative study of a ward in a house. In Wing, J. K. (ed.) Long-Term Community Care: experience in a London borough. *Psychological Medicine*, Monograph Supplement No. 2. Cambridge: Cambridge University Press.

Table of cases

Bratty v AG for Northern Ireland (1963) AC 386.
Knight v Home Office (1990) *The Independent* 24 January
R v Birch (1989) 11 Cr App R (S) 202.
R v Castro (1985) 81 Cr App R (S) 212 CA.
R v Clarke (1972) 1 All ER 219; (1972) 56 Cr App R 225 CA.
R v Gunnell (1966) 50 Cr App R 242 CA.
R v Hennessy (1989) 1 WLR 287 CA.
R v Kaye (1988) The Times 25 May.
R v Mersey Mental Health Review Tribunal Ex p Dillon, 19 March 1986, *The Times* 13 April 1987.
R v M'Naghten (1843) 10 Cl & Fin 200.
R v The Nottingham Mental Health Review Tribunal Ex p Secretary of State for the Home Department (Thomas), 15 September 1988.
R v Quick (1973) QB 910.
R v Trent Mental Health Review Tribunal Ex p Secretary of State for the Home Department, 15 September 1988.
Re Golden Chemical Products Ltd (1976) Ch 300.
R v Sullivan (1984) AC 156.
Secretary of State for the Home Department v Mental Health Review Tribunal for the Mersey Regional Health Authority (1986) 1 WLR 1170.
Waldron, Re (1985) 3 WLR 1090.

Index